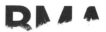

An Introduction to
Pharmacovigilance

An Introduction to Pharmacovigilance

Second Edition

Patrick Waller
Formerly Honorary Professor,
London School of Hygiene and Tropical Medicine,
London, United Kingdom

Mira Harrison-Woolrych
Honorary Research Associate Professor,
Dunedin School of Medicine, University of Otago,
New Zealand; Senior Medical Assessor, Vigilance and Risk
Management, Medicines and Healthcare products Regulatory
Agency (MHRA), London, United Kingdom and Secretary General
of the International Society of Pharmacovigilance (ISoP)

WILEY Blackwell

This edition first published 2017. © 2017 John Wiley & Sons Ltd
First edition published 2010 by John Wiley & Sons Ltd

Wiley-Blackwell is an imprint of John Wiley & Sons, formed by the merger of Wiley's global Scientific, Technical and Medical business with Blackwell Publishing.

Registered Office
John Wiley & Sons Ltd, The Atrium, Southern Gate, Chichester, West Sussex, PO19 8SQ, UK

Editorial Offices
9600 Garsington Road, Oxford, OX4 2DQ, UK
The Atrium, Southern Gate, Chichester, West Sussex, PO19 8SQ, UK
111 River Street, Hoboken, NJ 07030-5774, USA

For details of our global editorial offices, for customer services and for information about how to apply for permission to reuse the copyright material in this book please see our website at www.wiley.com/wiley-blackwell.

Library of Congress Cataloging-in-Publication Data

Names: Waller, Patrick, 1957 January 30– author. | Harrison-Woolrych, Mira, author.
Title: An introduction to pharmacovigilance / Patrick Waller, Mira Harrison-Woolrych.
Description: 2nd edition. | Chichester, West Sussex, UK ; Hoboken, NJ : John Wiley & Sons Inc., [2017] | Includes bibliographical references and index.
Identifiers: LCCN 2016059298| ISBN 9781119289746 (pbk.) | ISBN 9781119289753 (Adobe PDF) | ISBN 9781119289784 (epub)
Subjects: | MESH: Pharmacovigilance | Drug Monitoring–methods | Drug-Related Side Effects and Adverse Reactions | Pharmaceutical Preparations–standards
Classification: LCC RM302.5 | NLM QV 771 | DDC 615/.7042–dc23
   LC record available at https://lccn.loc.gov/2016059298

A catalogue record for this book is available from the British Library.

Cover Design: Wiley
Cover Credit: © Jorg Greuel/Gettyimages

Set in 10/12pt Warnock by SPi Global, Pondicherry, India
Printed and bound in Malaysia by Vivar Printing Sdn Bhd

10 9 8 7 6 5 4 3 2 1

The book is dedicated to the memory of the late Dr Susan M. Wood, an inspirational person who worked tirelessly in the field of pharmacovigilance for 10 years before her premature death in 1998.

About the authors

Patrick Waller was an Honorary Professor at the London School of Hygiene and Tropical Medicine 2011–2016 and Chair of the Independent Scientific Advisory Committee (ISAC) for Medicines and Healthcare products Regulatory Agency (MHRA) database research 2012–2016. He graduated in medicine in Sheffield, and then trained in clinical pharmacology and public health. Subsequently he worked at the Drug Safety Research Unit in Southampton and the Medicines Control Agency in London. He was Chairman of the EU Pharmacovigilance Working Party 1998–2000 and an independent consultant in pharmacovigilance and pharmacoepidemiology 2002–2011.

Mira Harrison-Woolrych is an Honorary Research Associate Professor at the Dunedin School of Medicine, University of Otago. With a background in clinical obstetrics and gynaecology, she has over 20 years' experience in pharmacovigilance in both the UK and New Zealand. She is currently Secretary General of the International Society of Pharmacovigilance (ISoP). As a Senior Medical Assessor at the UK MHRA, Mira specialises in women's medicines and in 2015 edited the textbook *Medicines for Women*. Between 2003 and 2013, she was the Director of the NZ Intensive Medicines Monitoring Programme (IMMP) and has an extensive list of pharmacoepidemiology research publications. She has also served on several national and international pharmacovigilance committees.

Contents

Foreword

No effective medicine is without risk, and full understanding of a medicine's safety profile is only achieved after wide clinical use. The advent of new therapies which hold the promise of transforming disease outlook means that patients and healthcare professionals are unwilling to wait to access them. It also means that the uncertainties around the balance of benefits and risks at the time of first availability of a new medicine may be greater than ever.

With every therapeutic advance, the boundaries between categories of healthcare products – medicines, advanced therapies, diagnostic agents – become ever more blurred and the practice of medicine more personalised to the individual patient. The continuing need for the study of medicines safety in wider populations could perhaps be called into question.

In fact, the study of drug safety in clinical use has moved to centre stage in public health, precisely because of the recognition that although by and large adverse effects are rare, it is only by undertaking systematic large-scale surveillance that we can detect serious problems early and take prompt action to minimise harms – as it were, to 'fix it while you fly'.

Pharmaceuticals are used internationally and the need for effective drug safety monitoring is recognised worldwide. A signal of a safety issue associated with a new medicine introduced in a public health programme in a resource-limited setting is just as relevant to a patient who may receive the same medicine in a high-tech healthcare environment. The political landscape may shift, but pharmacovigilance knows no borders.

The detection and evaluation of adverse effects associated with medicines involves specialists from a range of scientific disciplines who are attracted by the challenges of adding new knowledge that supports safe use of medicines. But pharmacovigilance can only be effective if it is relevant to the daily lives and embedded in the professional practice of all those who use medicines – the prescriber, the patient and their carer. There is clear evidence that reports from patients provide invaluable information on the impact of an adverse effect on life and work, and are of an equivalent level of seriousness to those from healthcare professionals.

This all adds up to the value of a broad appreciation and an up-to-date understanding of the principles and practice of pharmacovigilance. This new edition of a clear and succinct yet comprehensive guide to the field provides exactly the right introduction for those new to the challenges and the excitement of pharmacovigilance. It conveys the importance to public health protection of an effective safety net to pick up new information, and the need for well-planned strategies to generate new evidence as an enabler of innovation.

Everyone who uses a medicine has a part to play in helping to fill the knowledge gaps on safety in as near to real-time as possible. While pharmacovigilance has now moved on to more robust forms of evidence than reliance on individual case reports of adverse effects, the alert prescriber or patient who observes a possible link between a medicine they are using and an adverse effect is still the cornerstone of pharmacovigilance. The appreciation that each one of us has a role in drug safety means that this updated book is not only a welcome but an essential guide.

Dr June Raine CBE
Director of Vigilance and Risk Management of Medicines
Medicines and Healthcare Products Regulatory Agency, London, UK
and Chair of the EU Pharmacovigilance Risk Assessment Committee

Preface to the Second Edition

The general aim of this book – to provide a brief and broad introduction for newcomers to the field which can be read through in a few hours – has not changed since publication of the first edition in early 2010. In this second edition, we have updated every chapter to reflect pharmacovigilance practice in mid-2016 and have also broadened its international scope. Pharmacovigilance today is a global activity and our aim is to provide a short introduction relevant to readers worldwide. In response to feedback received on the first edition, we have added a new chapter on clinical aspects of pharmacovigilance (Chapter 7), which we hope will help readers without a medical background understand the importance of drug safety in 'real life'. For reference, we have added a list of all the abbreviations used in the book and we have also considerably expanded the glossary.

All scientific books are at risk of rapidly becoming out of date. When this one was first published, major changes in the landscape of regulatory pharmacovigilance were already in progress, particularly in the European Union (EU). During the intervening years, these changes have come into force and bedded down (see Chapter 5). In June 2016, the UK electorate voted to leave the EU and the full implications of 'Brexit' are not yet clear. However, the need for international collaboration in pharmacovigilance will not diminish and we expect that the worldwide networks discussed in Chapter 6 will be more important than ever before.

We hope that the new edition of this book will prove useful to those entering this interesting and important field. Life may have moved on, but the challenges involved in monitoring the safety of medicines – and taking effective action to protect patients from harm – remain as great as ever.

Patrick Waller, UK
Mira Harrison-Woolrych, New Zealand
September 2016

Preface to the First Edition

Everyone knows that safety is important but, apart from a few people whose job it is to oversee safety, this is probably something that most people have at the back of their minds for most of the time. There are likely to be two reasons for this – first, safety is about something adverse not happening (and we tend to be more concerned about things which are happening) and, secondly, it seems to be human nature to think that 'it will not happen to me', perhaps as a mechanism for coping with potential threat of something devastating.

The past decade has seen a marked rise in the numbers of people working in the field of clinical drug safety or pharmacovigilance, mostly in the pharmaceutical industry. The trend seems likely to continue, hopefully reflecting a greater focus on the safety of medicines. This book is specifically targeted at newcomers to the field who, of necessity, are often narrowly focused, and it aims to provide them with a brief and broad introduction to the field. My purpose here is to aid rapid understanding of the environment and key principles of pharmacovigilance at the industry–regulatory interface.

My background is in regulation and my experience is of the UK and EU systems and I readily acknowledge these inherent biases in my narrative. This book probably will not help the newcomers with detailed day-to-day aspects of their job but I hope it will enable them to see where they fit into a bigger picture. I have assumed that readers will at least have a science degree but not necessarily much specific knowledge about drugs.

The new entrant needs to know how we got where we are today. The most important historical drug safety issues have shaped the development of pharmacovigilance and I have therefore used these as a starting point. I hope that the book will also help the newcomers to appreciate that they are now working in an interesting and important field that is likely to develop much in the near future.

I have deliberately not included any reference citations within the text since, initially, I hope the reader will want to read on rather than go elsewhere. Ample references can be found in the larger texts on to which the reader should next move. In the last chapter, I have selectively cited some important sources that might usefully be consulted for further reading. A glossary defining key terms is provided at the end for reference.

Patrick Waller

Acknowledgements

We are most grateful to Ian Boyd and Nourieh Hoveyda who provided valuable comments on the whole redrafted manuscript for this edition. We are also grateful to the following people for review of specific chapters and useful suggestions: Priya Bahri, Keith Beard, Stephen Evans, Valerie Joynson, Marie Lindquist, Julie Williams and Jonathan Woolrych. We would also like to thank the Medicines and Healthcare products Regulatory Agency for providing data from the Yellow Card scheme.

List of Abbreviations

ACE	angiotensin converting enzyme
ADR	adverse drug reaction
AE	adverse event
ATC	Anatomical Therapeutic Chemical (classification system)
CIOMS	Council for International Organizations of Medical Sciences
COX	cyclo-oxygenase
CSM	Committee on Safety of Medicines
CTD	Common Technical Document
CYP450	cytochrome P450
DIA	Drug Information Association
DoTS	dose-relatedness, time course and susceptibility
DSRU	Drug Safety Research Unit
DSUR	Development Safety Update Report
EBGM	empirical Bayes geometric mean
ECG	electrocardiogram
EMA	European Medicines Agency
ENCePP	European Network of Centres for Pharmacoepidemiology and Pharmacovigilance
ESoP	European Society of Pharmacovigilance (now ISoP)
ESTRI	Electronic Standards for the Transfer of Regulatory Information
EU2P	European Programme in Pharmacovigilance and Pharmacoepidemiology
FDA	Food and Drug Administration
2G	second generation (oral contraceptive)
3G	third generation (oral contraceptive)

GP	general practitioner
GVP	good pharmacovigilance practice
HRT	hormone replacement therapy
IBD	international birth date
IC	information component
ICH	International Council (formerly Conference) on Harmonisation of Technical Requirements for Pharmaceuticals for Human Use
ICMRA	International Coalition of Medicines Regulatory Authorities
IMMP	Intensive Medicines Monitoring Programme
ISoP	International Society of Pharmacovigilance
ISPE	International Society for Pharmacoepidemiology
MA	marketing authorisation
MedDRA	Medical Dictionary for Regulatory Activities
MGPS	Multi-Item Gamma Poisson Shrinker
MHRA	Medicines and Healthcare products Regulatory Agency
MHT	menopausal hormone therapy
MMR	measles, mumps and rubella (vaccine)
NOAC	novel oral anticoagulant
NSAID	non-steroidal anti-inflammatory drug
OC	oral contraceptive
OTC	over-the-counter (medicine)
PASS	post-authorisation safety study
PBRER	Periodic Benefit–Risk Evaluation Report
PEM	prescription-event monitoring
PIDM	Programme for International Drug Monitoring
PIL	Patient Information Leaflet
PPAR	peroxisome proliferator-activated receptor
PRAC	Pharmacovigilance Risk Assessment Committee
PRR	proportional reporting ratio
PSUR	Periodic Safety Update Report
QPPV	qualified person for pharmacovigilance
RMP	risk management plan
ROR	reporting odds ratio
SAMM	Safety Assessment of Marketed Medicines
SIG	special interest group
SJS	Stevens–Johnson syndrome
SPC (or SmPC)	Summary of Product Characteristics

SSRI	selective serotonin re-uptake inhibitor
SUSAR	serious and unexpected suspected adverse reaction
TEN	toxic epidermal necrolysis
TGA	Therapeutic Goods Administration
UMC	Uppsala Monitoring Centre
UNESCO	United Nations Educational, Scientific and Cultural Organization
VTE	venous thromboembolism
WHO	World Health Organization
WHO-ART	World Health Organization Adverse Reaction Terminology
WHO-PIDM	World Health Organization Programme for International Drug Monitoring
WMA	World Medical Association

1

What is Pharmacovigilance and How Has it Developed?

Origins and Definition of Pharmacovigilance

In the beginning, there was thalidomide. The history of drug safety goes back further but, for practical purposes, the story of modern pharmacovigilance begins there.

In the late 1950s there was little, if any, regulation of medicines outside the USA (where thalidomide was not allowed on to the market), and their testing and development was almost entirely in the hands of pharmaceutical companies. In the case of thalidomide, unjustified claims of safety in pregnancy were made, and its use as a sedative and treatment for nausea and vomiting was targeted at pregnant women. The drug turned out to be a teratogen, producing a variety of birth defects but particularly limb defects known as phocomelia (Figure 1.1). Worldwide, about 10 000 babies were affected, particularly in Germany where the drug was first marketed. As phocomelia was otherwise a very rare congenital abnormality, a major increase in its incidence did not go unnoticed in Germany, but the cause was initially thought to be environmental. In 1961, a series of just three cases of congenital anomalies associated with thalidomide use in Australia was reported in *The Lancet*, the problem was finally recognised and the drug withdrawn from sale.

At the beginning of the 1960s, publication of possible adverse effects of drugs in the medical literature was effectively the only mechanism for drawing attention to them. Thalidomide produced a non-lethal but visible and shocking adverse effect, leading people to ask why so many damaged babies had been born before anything had been done? This question is central to subsequent developments. It is unlikely that we

An Introduction to Pharmacovigilance, Second Edition. Patrick Waller and Mira Harrison-Woolrych.
© 2017 John Wiley & Sons Ltd. Published 2017 by John Wiley & Sons Ltd.

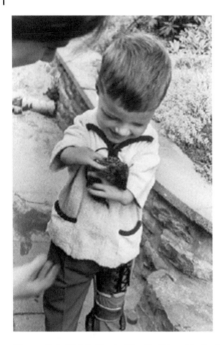

Figure 1.1 Child affected by thalidomide-induced phocomelia.

will ever be able to predict and prevent all the harms that may be caused by medicines, but limiting the damage to much smaller numbers is now achievable. Today we would expect to be able to identify an association between drug and outcome analogous to thalidomide and phocomelia after the occurrence of less than 10 cases, so at least three orders of magnitude more effectively than six decades ago.

The overriding lesson learnt from thalidomide was that we cannot just wait until a drug safety problem hits us. The thalidomide tragedy of the 1960s led directly to the initial development of the systems we have in place today, although it is only since the early 1990s that the term pharmacovigilance has become widely accepted.

Pharmacovigilance is defined by the World Health Organization as 'The science and activities relating to the detection, assessment, understanding and prevention of adverse effects or any other drug-related problems.' There are other definitions but this very broad one seems to be the most appropriate because there is a clear implication that the process is one of risk management. This is a concept that is applicable to many aspects of modern life but, surprisingly, its explicit use in relation to pharmaceuticals is a fairly recent development. Thalidomide is not merely of historical interest, as in recent years it has made a comeback on to the market in some countries but with very narrow indications and extensive safeguards. The reasons for this exemplify the point about risk management, as the risk of fetal malformation can be successfully managed by avoidance of the drug during pregnancy. It also demonstrates another concept that is central to the practice of pharmacovigilance – the balance of benefit and risk. Thalidomide has benefits in some diseases that are otherwise difficult to treat (e.g. refractory multiple myeloma) and these appear to outweigh the risk of fetal malformation if there is an effective pregnancy prevention scheme in place. A further point that thalidomide illustrates well – and which is relevant to many other drug safety issues – is that not everyone is at the same risk of a particular adverse effect. In this case, a substantial part of the population (including men and also women who are not of childbearing capacity) are not at risk of phocomelia.

Main Lessons Learned from Thalidomide

The thalidomide tragedy taught us many lessons:

- The need for adequate testing of medicines prior to marketing.
- The need for government regulation of medicines.
- The need for reporting systems to *identify* the adverse effects of medicines.
- The potential safety implications of unproven marketing claims.
- Most medicines cross the placenta and this results in fetal exposure.
- Avoidance of unnecessary use of medicines in pregnancy.
- That some risks can be successfully minimised.

The ramifications of the thalidomide tragedy were manyfold, but the key lesson for the development of pharmacovigilance was that active systems for detecting hazards are needed. Within a few years this had been taken forward with the introduction of voluntary (or 'spontaneous') schemes for reporting of suspected adverse drug reactions (ADRs). These have stood the test of time as an alerting mechanism or early warning system, and are covered in more detail in Chapter 3.

Scope and Purposes of Pharmacovigilance

In the past, the process of pharmacovigilance has often been considered to start when a drug is first authorised for use in ordinary practice. Nowadays, it is more commonly considered to include all safety-related activity beyond the point at which humans are first exposed to a new medicinal product.

The ultimate purpose of pharmacovigilance is to minimise, in practice, the potential for harm that is associated with all active medicines. Although data about all types of ADRs are collected, a key focus is on identifying and preventing those that are defined to be *serious*. This is generally defined as an ADR that meets at least one of the following criteria:

- Fatal
- Life-threatening
- Causes or prolongs hospitalisation
- Results in long-term disability
- All congenital anomalies.

The definition of serious also allows the application of medical judgement, such that a reaction can be considered serious even if there is not clear evidence that one of the above criteria is met. Non-serious reactions are important to individual patients and health professionals involved in their treatment, but they can usually be managed clinically and impact less on the balance of benefit and risk for individual products and on public health in general.

Thus, pharmacovigilance can be seen as a public health function in which reductions in the occurrence of serious harms are achievable through measures that promote the safest possible use of medicinal products and/or provide specific safeguards against known hazards. Pregnancy prevention in users of thalidomide is an example of such a safeguard; monitoring white blood cell counts to detect agranulocytosis (absent white blood cells) in users of the antipsychotic drug clozapine is another (see Chapter 7).

In order to minimise harms, there is first a need to identify and assess the impact of unexpected potential hazards. For most medicines, serious ADRs are rare, otherwise their detection would result in the drug not reaching (or being withdrawn from) the market. For products that do reach the market, serious hazards are seldom identified during pre-marketing clinical trials because sample sizes are invariably too small to detect them. In addition, the prevailing conditions of clinical trials – selected patients, short durations of treatment, close monitoring and specialist supervision – usually mean that the frequency of ADRs will be underestimated relative to what will really occur in ordinary practice.

During pre-marketing clinical development and research on new medicines, the aims of pharmacovigilance are rather different from the broad public health functions described here. In volunteer studies and clinical trials, there is a need to protect individuals exposed to experimental products (from which they may derive no benefit) from potential harm. There is also a need to gather information on risks (including the frequencies at which they happen) in order to make a provisional assessment of safety and to plan for post-marketing safety development (see Risk Management Planning in Chapter 5).

Development of Pharmacovigilance

We next consider some of the most important examples of drug safety issues and discuss how they have affected the development of pharmacovigilance practice from the 1960s to the present day.

Practolol

In the early 1970s another drug safety disaster occurred; this was the oculo-mucocutaneous syndrome, a multi-system disorder, caused by practolol (Eraldin), a cardioselective beta-blocker used to treat angina and hypertension. As in the case of thalidomide, several thousand individuals were permanently damaged before the association was recognised. The fundamental problem in this instance was a failure of timely identification, as despite having an early warning system in place, the system was dependent on doctors suspecting an association between drug and disease. Probably because of the unusual nature of the syndrome – dry eyes, skin rash and bowel obstruction – and a long latency period (averaging almost 2 years in respect of the onset of the most serious bowel manifestations), relevant cases were not reported until the association was identified in the medical literature. Around 3000 cases were then retrospectively reported to the UK Yellow Card spontaneous ADR reporting scheme (see Chapter 3), an example of the potential effect of publicity on ADR reporting. Interestingly, subsequent attempts to develop an animal model of practolol toxicity failed, indicating that the problem could not have been predicted from pre-clinical studies.

Main Lessons Learned from Practolol
- Some adverse effects are not predictable from pre-clinical studies.
- Spontaneous reporting schemes are not always effective at identifying new ADRs.
- Health professionals may not be able to identify long latency effects and clinical manifestations not known to be related to other drugs as ADRs.
- Additional, proactive and more systematic methods of studying post-marketing safety are needed.

The overriding message from practolol was that spontaneous ADR reporting alone is insufficient as a means of studying post-marketing safety. Thus, in the late 1970s various schemes designed to closely monitor the introduction of new drugs were suggested, but few implemented. The basic idea was that initial users of new drugs would be identified through prescriptions and monitored systematically rather than waiting for someone to recognise a possible adverse effect. The concept did come to fruition in New Zealand and in England in the late 1970s with the development of nationwide prescription-event monitoring (PEM) programmes (see Chapter 3).

Benoxaprofen

The first drug studied by PEM in England was benoxaprofen (Opren), a non-steroidal anti-inflammatory drug (NSAID) which frequently produced photosensitivity reactions (i.e. rashes in light-exposed areas). A published case series from Northern Ireland of five deaths related to hepatic and renal failure led to withdrawal of the drug in 1982, although the PEM study did not reveal any indication of these effects. Many of the patients who experienced serious ADRs with benoxaprofen were elderly; this was a result of reduced excretion of the drug as a consequence of renal impairment. Even though it is well-recognised that many patients who use NSAIDs are elderly (e.g. for arthritis or chronic pain), benoxaprofen had not been adequately studied in this population prior to marketing. A reduction in the dosage recommendations for the elderly was implemented briefly, but benoxaprofen was withdrawn soon afterwards.

Because the usage of benoxaprofen took off rapidly after launch and an important adverse effect – photosensitivity reactions – was common, a large number of spontaneous reports were received in a short period of time, swamping the primitive computer systems then used and pointing to the need for purpose-designed databases. The issue also illustrated the need for patients to be properly informed about possible ADRs and how to minimise the risk – in this case by avoiding exposure to the sun. It was therefore influential in moving towards the introduction of patient information leaflets, which became compulsory in the European Union (EU) during the 1990s.

Main Lessons Learned from Benoxaprofen

- Uncertainty about cause and effect from individual case reports – further impetus to the need for formal post-marketing studies in patient cohorts of sufficient size.
- The need to study a drug in populations most likely to use it (e.g. the elderly).
- The need for purpose-designed computer systems to handle ADR reports more promptly and effectively.
- The concept of intensive surveillance of new drugs, later achieved in the UK by the introduction of the Black Triangle scheme (see Glossary).
- The need for patients to be informed about possible ADRs.

Benoxaprofen was just the first of a series of NSAIDs withdrawn for various safety reasons in the 1980s. During this decade, pharmaceutical companies started to conduct their own post-marketing surveillance studies and UK guidelines related to their conduct were drawn up in 1987. However, initially, the value of such studies turned out to be limited because they usually lacked comparator groups and often failed to meet the planned sample size. The UK guidelines were revised in 1993 with the aim of improving the quality of studies. The principles of the revised Safety Assessment of Marketed Medicines (SAMM) guidelines also became a blueprint for the first EU level guidance on the topic.

Development of Pharmacoepidemiology

Epidemiology is the study of the distribution and determinants of health and disease in populations. During the mid-1980s, the term pharmacoepidemiology was first used to mean the scientific discipline of the study of drug use and safety at a population level. The discipline developed strongly during the 1990s with the increasing use of computerised databases containing records of prescriptions and clinical outcomes for rapid and efficient study of potential safety hazards. In some instances, prescription records are held in a separate database to clinical events, and linkage between the two databases needs to be achieved (through common identifiers in the two sets of data) in order to study adverse events at an individual patient level.

Towards the end of the 1980s, pharmacovigilance and pharmacoepidemiology started to investigate the problem of dependence on benzodiazepines – so-called minor tranquillisers such as chlordiazepoxide (Librium) and diazepam (Valium) which had been introduced in the 1960s. Advice was issued to limit the dosage and duration of such treatments and this issue brought into focus the problems faced in dealing with the misuse and abuse of prescription drugs. This is another example of a situation where spontaneous ADR reporting failed to highlight an important concern, the issue eventually coming into focus as a result of pressure from advocates for groups of affected patients.

As well as the problem of delayed identification of real hazards, pharmacovigilance has suffered from the reverse, the apparent identification of hazards that turn out not to be real. To some extent this is inherent in a system that relies much on clinical suspicions – sometimes these will be wrong. The consequences are that sometimes a drug is unnecessarily withdrawn, or people become too scared to use it. For example, Debendox (or Bendectin), a combination product containing the antihistamine doxylamine, was widely used for the treatment of nausea and vomiting in pregnancy in the 1970s. It was withdrawn in the early 1980s on the basis of concerns that it might cause fetal malformations, a concerted campaign against the drug and impending litigation. At the time, the evidence of a hazard was very weak, but it was not possible to exclude a significant risk to the fetus. Subsequently, many studies of this potential association were performed and, collectively, they provided no evidence of an increased risk of fetal malformations. This example illustrates the intrinsic difficulty of disproving the existence of a hazard once concern has been raised.

A more recent, very high profile example illustrating the same point was the suggestion made in late 1990s that the combined measles, mumps and rubella (MMR) vaccine might be a cause of autism in children.

Despite there being little evidence for this suggestion, it was impossible to completely disprove and hard to convince worried parents. Some years later the paper that provoked this concern was discredited and retracted but in the meantime vaccine campaigns were damaged and a significant number of cases of measles occurred in the UK for the first time in many years.

Oral Contraceptives and 'Pill Scares'

This major pharmacovigilance story began in the late 1960s when it was discovered through spontaneous ADR reporting – and later confirmed in formal studies – that combined oral contraceptives (OCs) (containing an estrogen and a progestogen) increased the risk of venous thromboembolism (VTE). This led to a reduction in the dose of estrogen to 20–30 μg ethinylestradiol, which lessened (but did not abolish) the risk without compromising efficacy. Nevertheless, when the risk of thrombosis became public knowledge (highlighted by media 'pill scare' stories in some countries), many women became very worried and stopped taking OCs. When OCs are stopped abruptly by sexually active women, without immediate use of an effective alternative, unintended pregnancies occur and rates of induced abortion increase.

There have been several 'pill scares' over the years related to VTE and also to other safety issues such as a possible association with myocardial infarction and a small increase in the risk of breast cancer. In each of these scares, many women stopped using OCs and the public health impact, in terms of unintended pregnancies, was considerable. This has been particularly unfortunate because pregnancy itself is riskier (with higher rates of VTE for example) than using any OC.

In 1995, a World Health Organization (WHO) study of OCs found a twofold increase in the risk of VTE when use of third-generation (3G) OCs was compared with second-generation (2G) OCs. The difference between these pills was the progestagen component; desogestrel or gestodene for 3G OCs and levonorgestrel for 2G OCs. This was surprising, as it had always been considered that VTE risk was simply related to the dose of estrogen in the pill. Within about 3 months of the WHO study, the results of two other studies reached similar conclusions. Arguments were put forward that the associations seen in these studies were not necessarily causal and that 3G

OCs might have benefits that would compensate for the increase in VTE risk. However, there was general agreement that although the *relative* risk of VTE was doubled with 3G pills, the *absolute* level of risk (see Chapter 2) was very low, as VTE is rare in healthy young women, even if they take the pill. Thus, there was general agreement that 3G OCs should not be withdrawn from the market.

The UK's Committee on Safety of Medicines (CSM) decided that the emerging information on VTE risk should be shared with doctors and patients, but faced several challenges around communicating the risks of the OC pill. Scare stories had already been published in the British press and despite CSM messages that no one should stop taking OCs, many women did, and hundreds of unintended pregnancies subsequently occurred. It seemed that women had acted on information provided by the mainstream media, rather than on advice provided by a national medicines advisory committee. Interestingly, the pill scare that occurred in the UK in 1995 was not seen in other countries, even those where use of OCs is high. There could be many reasons for this, including the role of the British press in risk communication.

Following the 1995 pill scare, more studies were carried out and the effects of the various progestagens on blood clotting investigated. Ultimately, it was shown that there were plausible differential effects of these agents on clotting and further pharmacoepidemiological studies have now convinced most scientists that the observed association was causal and that 2G pills have the lowest risk of VTE. It has also been acknowledged that the risk communication tools used in 1995 were inadequate and, in many respects, pharmacovigilance risk communication at that time failed to prevent serious public health outcomes. In 1997, the WHO convened a meeting of experts to consider how communication in pharmacovigilance could be improved (see Chapter 4). Since then, there have been other significant developments in risk communication for all medicinal products and many of these have been informed by lessons learned from OC pill scares.

Main Lessons Learned from the OC Safety Issues

- Drugs are sometimes marketed at a higher dose than is required for efficacy.
- There may be differences in safety between drugs of the same class.
- Harm can result from poor communication of safety warnings.

- When communicating risks of medicines, it is important to distinguish between relative and absolute risks (see Chapter 2) and to explain the difference in plain language.
- Uncertainty and debate about risks can fuel public concern.
- The power of the media to influence users may be greater than the authorities.
- The need for greater international cooperation in pharmacovigilance.
- The need to develop more effective communication tools.
- Risk communication is a specific skill in pharmacovigilance.

An important point about the OC issues discussed is that the data on which they were based did not, after the initial signal in the 1960s, come from spontaneous ADR reporting. Despite that, causation was debatable because the studies were not randomised trials but observational pharmacoepidemiology studies. VTE is a sufficiently rare outcome in young women that it would be extremely difficult to conduct a large enough randomized clinical trial to detect a doubling of risk.

Hormone Replacement Therapy (Menopausal Hormone Therapy)

Later in life, women have also been prescribed sex hormones as replacement therapy (HRT, now renamed menopausal hormone therapy; MHT). In this age group, the baseline risks of VTE, arterial cardiovascular disease and various cancers are much greater and therefore it has been more feasible to study them in clinical trials, although studies have needed to be large and long-term. Therefore, observational studies of these outcomes were performed first and, in general, they appeared to show that HRT *reduced* the risk of arterial disease outcomes such as myocardial infarction and stroke. HRT was never authorised for the purpose of reducing cardiovascular risk, but in the 1980s and 1990s, on the basis of results from observational studies and much pharmaceutical company promotion, it was widely used for this purpose. The fundamental problem in performing such studies is that women using HRT may be healthier to start with and it is difficult to address all possible *confounding* factors (see Glossary) in the design and analysis of observational studies. Another important point is that the outcome in question is a *benefit* (i.e. a reduction in risk) and, because of such *biases* (see Glossary), observational studies rarely provide convincing evidence of benefit. It is generally accepted that randomised trials are needed to establish efficacy and benefit.

Eventually, large randomised trials of HRT were set up (e.g. the Million Women Study), but some studies had to be stopped early because they showed the opposite of what was expected – an *increase* in cardiovascular risk. Warnings were then issued by regulatory authorities and, because there is no major downside to suddenly stopping HRT, communication was intrinsically easier than with OCs. Indeed, the intended effect of the warnings was that women who were inappropriately using long-term HRT should stop taking it. However, conveying the right messages was not straightforward because there were multiple risks involved, and they are time-dependent and cannot simply be expressed as a proportion (e.g. 1 in 100). In 2007, the UK authorities published a report on HRT which included estimates of risk for several adverse outcomes, expressed in clear language. Since then, further studies of HRT have been published and discussion of the risks and benefits of these products continues, and is likely to for some time to come.

Selective Serotonin Re-uptake Inhibitors

Selective serotonin re-uptake inhibitors (SSRIs) are antidepressants which were brought to the market in the late 1980s and have since largely replaced older, tricyclic antidepressants such as amitriptyline. The main reason why they have done so – apart from effective marketing – is that they are less toxic to the heart in overdose (i.e. there is a greater margin of safety in relation to dose). Depressed patients are at risk of taking an overdose and therefore this is potentially an important advantage.

There have been two controversial issues with SSRIs: withdrawal reactions and a possible increase in the risk of suicide. Problems experienced by patients when they stop treatments are often quite difficult to assess because they could possibly be related to recurrence of the disease. Nevertheless, the potential for SSRIs to produce withdrawal reactions was identified during their development, and when spontaneous reports were received post-marketing it was hardly a new *signal* (see Glossary). There were very large numbers of such reports received, but few were serious and the level of usage of the drugs was high. Over a period of years it became clear that the problem was occurring much more commonly than initially thought, particularly in users of paroxetine (Seroxat), a fairly short-acting drug. Ultimately, greater care was needed in withdrawing patients more gradually from these drugs. Suggestions have been made that SSRIs are drugs of dependence but most scientists do not accept this because features such as craving and dose-escalation are generally absent. Importantly, it emerged that the nature of some of the more unpleasant symptoms patients experienced – such as 'electric shock' sensations in the head – was being lost in the data processing systems. This was often a result of inadequate coding. Such cases often became 'paraesthesia' (a tingling or prickling sensation), something that hardly conveys how unpleasant such sensations can be. Thus, it was recognised that we needed better ways to capture unusual patient experiences and this gave considerable impetus to allowing patients to report their adverse reactions to the authorities. That approach had been used in the USA and some other countries for many years, but hardly at all in Europe until the early years of the twenty-first century.

The possibility that any drug might increase the risk of an outcome associated with the disease it is being used to treat is invariably difficult to evaluate. Suicidal feelings and actions are relatively common in depressed patients and it is not surprising when they occur in a patient who has recently started treatment. Nevertheless, around 1990, a clinician in the USA saw several patients treated with fluoxetine (Prozac) who had suicidal thoughts and he published a case series suggesting that the drug might be responsible. This prompted a review of all the clinical trial data for the drug which did not support the proposition, but it was never completely refuted.

Over the years more clinical trial data accumulated for various drugs in the class and studies were conducted in children and adolescents, the latter being a high-risk group for suicide. Even in severely depressed patients, completed suicides are rare in clinical trials and therefore the evidence available relates mostly to attempted suicide (also uncommon in trials) and thoughts of suicide measured on various scales. Trials of paroxetine in children produced adverse findings – an increased risk of suicidal behaviour and hostility – which for some time were known only to the manufacturer. When the regulatory authorities eventually received the data, they issued warnings against the use of this drug in children. The company was investigated and prosecution considered, but the law was found to be insufficiently clear that the company was obliged to submit concerning clinical trial data immediately to the authorities when a trial was being conducted outside the authorised indication. Again, this issue pointed to the potential importance of clinical trials in the assessment of safety and raised concern about a lack of transparency with clinical trial data. Considerable steps have since been taken towards making clinical trial data publicly available through mechanisms other than publication in the literature which is slow and selective. There is still some uncertainty as to whether SSRIs directly increase the risk of suicide in adults, but there is general agreement that the early phase of treatment is a high-risk period and that careful monitoring of patients is required.

COX-2 Inhibitors

What have been the most prominent drug safety issues of the twenty-first century? One of the most important has been the increased risk of cardiovascular outcomes associated with selective COX-2 inhibitors (coxibs). This possibility was first uncovered in basic research but not followed through. The first clinical indication of a problem came from the VIGOR trial which was published in 2000. At the time, two drugs in the class – rofecoxib and celecoxib – had just been authorised. The VIGOR study was a randomised comparison of rofecoxib with naproxen (a standard NSAID), designed to establish whether there was a difference in the rates of serious gastrointestinal adverse effects (e.g. bleeding) of these two drugs. In that respect, rofecoxib was clearly preferable and the trial results led to rapid uptake of coxibs, on the basis that they were supposedly safer. However, the VIGOR study also found an important difference in the rate of cardiovascular events such as myocardial infarction which were five-fold more common in patients taking rofecoxib than with naproxen. This information was included in the original publication but lacked prominence and was presented as a fivefold reduction with naproxen rather than an increase with rofecoxib. The paper was subsequently the subject of extensive criticism.

Over the years there have been suggestions that standard NSAIDs reduce the risk of cardiovascular outcomes (as aspirin does) and a potential explanation for the finding in the VIGOR study put forward was that naproxen is cardioprotective whereas rofecoxib is not.

Ultimately, it took a large clinical trial comparing rofecoxib with placebo to establish beyond any doubt that this was an adverse effect of rofecoxib (rather than a lack of benefit) and the findings of that study led to the drug being withdrawn from the market in late 2004. This event sent shockwaves around the world leading people to question why such a trial had not been carried out much earlier, before millions of people had used the drug. It also left a big cloud hanging over the remaining drugs in the class; some were later withdrawn but some remain on the market. At one stage, the proposition that coxibs might be given to people at high risk of gastrointestinal bleeding and low risk of cardiovascular disease seemed reasonable, but it has since been discovered that, to a considerable extent, risk factors for these problems overlap in individual patients. To make matters even more complicated, it appears that some standard NSAIDs also increase the risk of cardiovascular events and the ability to assess the relative safety of drugs in the same class remains rather limited. This issue was a major driver of the considerable increase in post-marketing regulation, and focus on post-authorisation safety studies, which came to fruition in Europe in 2012 and is discussed in Chapter 5.

Two other notable drug safety issues of recent years are also important: the differing hazards associated with three glitazone drugs used to treat type 2 diabetes, and the association of pandemic flu vaccine with narcolepsy.

Glitazones

Troglitazone was the first of the three glitazones to be marketed in the late 1990s. These drugs are oral hypoglycaemics which work by activating peroxisome proliferator-activated receptors (PPARs). Soon after marketing, a considerable number of case reports of severe hepatotoxicity with associated liver failure were received and the drug was rapidly withdrawn in Europe. At the time, the next in class, rosiglitazone, was in the later stages of development and regulatory authorities therefore considered very carefully whether it might also be associated with a similar level of hepatotoxicity. They concluded (and were eventually proven right) that it was probably different in this regard. Rosiglitazone became a very widely used drug in the first few years of the twenty-first century and it was soon followed by pioglitazone. Studies of cardiovascular risk were performed with these drugs in the expectation that an effective anti-diabetic drug would reduce the risk. However, when these studies were brought together in a meta-analysis (which combines the results of multiple studies; see Chapter 3) published in 2007, the opposite appeared to be the case for rosiglitazone. This concern was the subject of considerable debate and further study but, within a couple of years, it led to the demise of the drug. Much of that debate was about its relative cardiovascular safety compared with pioglitazone.

Given that the benefits of the two drugs appeared broadly equal, and that most of the available evidence suggested that pioglitazone was safer, it was allowed to remain on the market. Interestingly, pioglitazone also appears to be associated with its own particular important safety problem, bladder cancer. This was originally identified in animal studies and in the last few years has been confirmed in humans. However, the level of risk is quite low, and considered manageable and to be outweighed by the benefits of the drug in effectively treating type 2 diabetes. The safety issues experienced with glitazones are remarkable. Despite the apparent similarities of the drugs, they appear to be associated with different important adverse effects affecting different organs.

Pandemrix

In 2009, there was an influenza pandemic reflecting the global spread of a new strain of human flu H1N1 virus. In many countries, mass vaccinations were undertaken with Pandemrix. In Finland and Sweden, case reports of a vaccinated children and adolescents developing narcolepsy – a brain disorder causing episodes of sudden onset of sleep at inappropriate times – were soon received. Formal studies have since confirmed this as a rare risk but only in young people, and the mechanism for this effect remains unclear. The effect has therefore been recognised in the product information and it has been recommended that this vaccine should no longer be used in patients under 20 years unless no other suitable vaccine is available. This example illustrates the effectiveness of the intensive ADR monitoring systems which were put in place to cover mass vaccinations during a pandemic in picking up an unusual and important adverse reaction.

Main Lessons Learned from Recent Major Safety Issues

- The need for vigorous follow-up of safety signals with appropriate studies.
- That drugs within the same class can have markedly different risks and the need for studies that address this possibility.
- The difficulty of assessing outcomes that are related to the drug indication.
- The potential value of randomized controlled clinical trials in assessing safety and the importance of the choice of comparator drug(s).
- Important safety data can emerge from clinical trials performed for other purposes.
- The need for greater transparency and increased availability of clinical trial data.
- The potential importance to safety of off-label use (e.g. in children).
- There is a need to evaluate medicines adequately in children and adolescents.
- The need for greater patient involvement in drug safety.
- The complexity of evaluating and communicating multiple risks (and benefits).
- The need for regulatory authorities to have sufficient powers to ensure that companies have adequate pharmacovigilance systems and proactively investigate potential risks with marketed products.

Conclusions

The issues discussed are necessarily selective and our discussion of them is broad. The intention is primarily to illustrate that pharmacovigilance experienced many teething problems in its early years and that most of its developments have been in response to quite specific lessons learned from landmark safety issues. In this chapter, we have tried to illustrate what pharmacovigilance is and, by describing important examples, how it has progressed over a period of more than half a century. Despite that progress, no one should doubt that there is still a long way to go. The current limitations of the discipline and how we might eventually overcome them are considered in Chapter 9.

2

Basic Concepts

The two most important concepts in pharmacovigilance are opposites: harm and safety. The usual term for harm related to a medicine is an adverse drug reaction (ADR). As pharmacovigilance is fundamentally about preventing and managing ADRs, this concept is considered first through a summary of relevant definitions, classification systems that have been proposed, their nature and mechanisms and predisposing factors. Subsequently, the concept of safety is defined and discussed, particularly in the context of balancing harms with benefits. Finally, we consider the issue of causation how we go about deciding whether or not a patient has experienced an ADR or whether a medicinal product really is responsible for an apparent safety problem.

Adverse Drug Reactions

Definitions

Standard, internationally agreed definitions of side effect, ADR and adverse event can be paraphrased as follows:

- A *side effect* is an *unintended effect of a medicine*. Normally, it is undesirable but it could be beneficial (e.g. an anxiolytic effect from a beta-blocker prescribed for hypertension).
- An *adverse drug reaction (ADR)* is an *unintended and noxious effect* that is attributable to a medicine when it has been given within the normal range of doses used in humans.

An Introduction to Pharmacovigilance, Second Edition. Patrick Waller and Mira Harrison-Woolrych.
© 2017 John Wiley & Sons Ltd. Published 2017 by John Wiley & Sons Ltd.

- An *adverse event (AE)* is an *undesirable occurrence* that occurs in the context of drug treatment but which *may or may not* be causally related to a medicine.

The difference between an ADR and an AE is crucial and yet these terms are widely misused. In practice, determining whether a drug is responsible for a particular AE in an individual patient is often difficult and a judgement has to be made (for an explanation of the principles on which this judgement is based see Causality Assessment in Individual Cases). When the judgement is that the drug is a possible cause, this should be called a *suspected ADR*. Reports of such suspicions form the basis of spontaneous ADR reporting schemes and the key point about such data is that they are a *subset* of all the AEs occurring during drug treatment which someone (generally a health professional who has seen the patient) has identified as possibly being drug-related. It is the clinician's experience and professional judgement that enables him or her to suspect a drug as the cause but, of course, that suspicion may not be correct.

Proper use of the term AE should imply that a more systematic data collection process has been used so that events will be included, regardless of whether anyone believes they might be caused by a drug. In most clinical trials it is a standard practice to document all AEs and the best way of determining whether a drug is responsible for a particular type of event from such data is by comparison with a control group. For example, if 10% of patients exposed to an active drug experienced headache compared to 2% on placebo, then this is an estimate that headache attributable to the drug occurs in 8% (i.e. 10% minus 2%) of patients using it. In such trials it is also common to ask investigators whether they believe that individual events are related to the drug. This is effectively another way of collecting suspected ADRs, although such data are likely to be more complete if the patient is in a clinical trial rather than being treated in ordinary practice. It is important to realise that relying on clinical judgement is a methodologically weaker approach. Providing that the estimated 8% difference is not based on very small numbers, then it would be more persuasive evidence that the drug causes headache.

Thus, the three terms should be applied in the following contexts:

- Use *ADR* to mean that it is now generally accepted that drug x may cause effect y rather than in relation to individual cases. Qualify the term with 'possible' if there is doubt.

- Use *suspected ADR* when a health professional or investigator indicates that a drug *may* have been responsible for an event in an individual case. A valid case submitted as a spontaneous report to a company or regulatory authority (see Chapter 5) is, by definition, a suspected ADR.
- Use *AE* only in the context of systematic data collection when no element of judgement is involved in determining whether a case is counted.

Classification Systems

Since the 1970s, ADRs have traditionally been classified into two broad categories: Types A and B. The usual characteristics of these different types of reactions are contrasted, followed by some examples:

1) *Type A* (Augmented) reactions are generally:
   - Dose-related
   - Predictable from drug pharmacology
   - Common
   - Reversible
   - Manageable with dose adjustment.

Classic examples of Type A reactions are bleeding with warfarin, hypoglycaemia with oral anti-diabetic agents and headache with nitrates.

2) *Type B* (Bizarre) reactions are generally:
   - Not dose-related
   - Unpredictable
   - Uncommon
   - Serious/irreversible
   - Indicative that the drug needs to be stopped.

Classic examples of Type B reactions are anaphylaxis with penicillins, hepatitis with halothane and agranulocytosis with clozapine.
   Additional categories of ADRs have also been suggested, as follows:

- Type C (Chronic), e.g. adrenal suppression with corticosteroids.
- Type D (Delayed), e.g. tardive dyskinesia with neuroleptics.
- Type E (End of use), e.g. withdrawal reactions with benzodiazepines.

DoTS Classification

In 2003, a system of classification was proposed by Aronson and Ferner based on *dose-relatedness, time course* and *susceptibility;* this is known as DoTS. The main ways in which ADRs can be classified within each of these three categories is given in Table 2.1.

In terms of dose-relatedness, 'toxic' means that reactions occur as a result of drug levels being too high, 'collateral' means that reactions occur at drug levels that are in the usual therapeutic range and 'hypersusceptibility' means that reactions can occur even at very low, sub-therapeutic doses. The terms 'early', 'intermediate' and 'late' have not been precisely defined; the main difference between 'late' and 'delayed' reactions is that the latter can occur long after treatment is stopped (e.g. cancer, which can occur years after exposure to a causal agent). A withdrawal reaction means one that is specifically precipitated by stopping the drug.

If suitable estimates of risk are available, it may be possible to draw three-dimensional DoTS diagrams of the probability of an ADR occurring in sub-groups over time and as a function of dose. When this is not possible, qualitative classification may still be useful, as shown by the following examples.

DoTS Classification: Examples

1) *Osteoporosis due to corticosteroids:* this reaction occurs at therapeutic doses, usually after some months of treatment. Females and older people are at the greatest risk. Hence, it would be classified as:

Table 2.1 Summary of dose-relatedness, time course and susceptibility (DoTS) categories.

Dose	Time	Susceptibility
Toxic	Independent	Age
Collateral	Dependent:	Gender
Hypersusceptibility	rapid administration	Ethnic origin
	first dose	Genetic
	early, intermediate, late	Disease
	delayed	
	withdrawal	

- Dose: collateral effect
- Time: late
- Susceptibility: age, sex.

2) *Anaphylaxis due to penicillin:* this reaction can occur with very small doses and within minutes of taking the first dose of a course, but true anaphylaxis only occurs when the drug (or a closely related agent) has been used previously. Hence, it would be classified as:
- Dose: hypersusceptibility
- Time: first dose
- Susceptibility: requires previous sensitisation.

The DoTS approach is useful because it addresses the limitations of the Type A/B scheme into which many ADRs do not clearly fit and in providing pointers as to how specific ADRs can be avoided.

Nature and Mechanisms of ADRs

The adverse effects of medicines usually mimic diseases or syndromes that occur naturally and have a variety of non-drug potential causes (e.g. hepatitis or aplastic anaemia). As a general rule, considering other potential causes is an important part of the assessment of a potential adverse effect (see Causality Assessment). However, there are a few unique syndromes that, as far as we yet know, seem to be caused only by specific drugs. Four examples of this are:

1) Vaginal cancer in young women caused by maternal exposure to diethylstilboestrol
2) Oculomucocutaneous syndrome caused by practolol (see Chapter 1)
3) Eosinophilia-myalgia syndrome caused by some L-tryptophan products
4) Fibrosing colonopathy induced by large doses of high-strength pancreatic enzymes in children with cystic fibrosis.

In broad terms, there are at least four mechanisms for ADRs:

1) Exaggerated therapeutic response at the target site (e.g. bleeding with warfarin)
2) Desired pharmacological effect at another site (e.g. headache with glyceryltrinitrate)
3) Additional (secondary) pharmacological actions (e.g. prolongation of the QT interval on the electrocardiogram – many drugs)
4) Triggering an immunological response (e.g. anaphylaxis due to many drugs).

Particularly at the time they are first identified, the mechanism of many ADRs is unknown or incompletely understood. Some have a pharmacokinetic basis e.g. impaired hepatic metabolism due to a genetic polymorphism or the effect of another medication taken concurrently, leading to increased plasma concentrations. Understanding genetic predispositions is likely to be an important factor in determining how we might prevent ADRs in the future (see Chapter 9).

Predisposing Factors for ADRs

The main clinical factors that increase the chance that patients will experience an adverse reaction are as follows:

- *Age* – the elderly and neonates are at greatest risk.
- *Gender* – women are generally at higher risk.
- *Ethnic origin* – can affect drug metabolism because of genetic predisposition.
- *Impaired excretory mechanisms* – reduced hepatic and/or renal function.
- *Specific diseases* – e.g. asthma and beta-blockers[1].
- *Polypharmacy* –use of multiple drugs simultaneously, increasing the potential for drug interactions (see next section).
- *Any previous history of an ADR.*

Drug Interactions

Drug interactions occur when the presence of one drug affects the activity of another. This occurs either because both drugs act through the same pathway(s) – these are called *pharmacodynamic* interactions – or through effects on absorption, distribution, metabolism or excretion – *pharmacokinetic* interactions. The result may be an adverse reaction or modified effectiveness. Some specific examples are given as follows:

- *Pharmacodynamic* – concomitant use of two drugs with similar effects. For example, an angiotensin converting enzyme (ACE) inhibitor plus a potassium-sparing diuretic can result in hyperkalaemia and cardiac arrhythmias.

---

[1] This is a very important example because the effect of beta-blockers in patients with asthma is to constrict the airways and to counteract some of the treatments that the patient may be taking (e.g. beta-agonists). Giving a beta-blocker to an asthmatic patient can prove to be fatal.

- *Absorption* – orlistat, a drug used to treat obesity, impairs the absorption of some medicines (e.g. anticonvulsants) and its use in this context could lead to convulsions.
- *Distribution* – protein-bound drugs (e.g. phenytoin, aspirin) can displace each other, resulting in an increased unbound (i.e. active) fraction of drug in plasma.
- *Metabolism* – many medicines (e.g. cimetidine and omeprazole), drugs that reduce gastric acid by different mechanisms, inhibit the metabolism of warfarin and thereby increase its anticoagulant effect, leading to bleeding reactions.
- *Excretion* – amiodarone, an anti-arrhythmic drug, reduces excretion of, and therefore the dosage requirements for, digoxin – a drug widely prescribed to patients with cardiac disease.

Many drugs are metabolised by hepatic cytochrome P450 (CYP450) enzymes, the activity of which may be induced or inhibited by a wide variety of drugs. There are several subgroups of CYP450 enzymes and their activity can also be affected by:

- *Herbal medicines* – e.g. St John's wort is an enzyme inducer and can reduce the effectiveness of various drugs including ciclosporin.
- *Dietary products* – e.g. grapefruit juice is an enzyme inhibitor and increases plasma concentrations of some calcium channel blockers, drugs that are used to treat hypertension and angina.

Drugs can also interact with *alcohol* – for example, metronidazole (an antibiotic) blocks part of the metabolic pathway for alcohol and concomitant use, which is not recommended, leads to intense vasodilatation.

The Concept of Safety

Definition

Safety can be defined as *relative absence of harm*. When using the word 'safety' we often mean something else. For example, safety data often means collection of reports of harm. Safety departments in the pharmaceutical industry are generally focused much more on harm than safety. And yet how safe something is a key question for the user and one that pharmacovigilance is gradually becoming more targeted at. To establish safety, it is not enough to sit around and hope that nothing much happens. Active processes are required to generate data in large numbers of users – this is one of the main challenges facing people working in the field.

In practice, there is no such thing as absolute safety because, even if something is completely harmless, it is impossible to demonstrate that with complete certainty. For example, if a drug were given to 999 999 people without any problem occurring, it would be very unlikely that the millionth person to use it would be harmed, but it is not impossible. In any case, we know that all pharmacologically active substances have the potential to cause harm. When we say that a drug is 'safe', we mean that there is a low probability of harm which, *in the context of the disease being treated and the expected benefits of the drug*, can be considered acceptable. Disease context is important because patients with more serious illnesses are much more likely to be prepared to accept potentially harmful treatments than those who have minor or self-limiting illnesses. 'Acceptability' is a subjective judgement which ultimately is made by comparing both the positive and the negative consequences of one course of action (e.g. a drug) with another (which could be any form of treatment or no treatment). We will return to this point in more detail in the section on risk–benefit balance.

Safety is a moving ball – there is a need to re-evaluate it as experience accumulates. Treatments previously considered acceptably safe may become 'unsafe' in the light of new evidence or the discovery of safer alternatives. An example of the latter was the antihistamine terfenadine which was widely used in the treatment of hay fever until the early 1990s. It was then discovered that it could, very rarely, cause serious or fatal ventricular arrhythmias through the mechanism of prolonging the QT interval. Terfenadine is a pro-drug (i.e. precursor of the active substance) which is normally completely metabolised on the first-pass through the liver. It is the parent drug terfenadine that prolongs the QT interval (when its metabolism is inhibited) but the metabolite is responsible for the beneficial effects. Thus, the metabolite, known as fexofenadine, was developed for this indication and rapidly accepted to be a safer alternative, following which terfenadine became obsolete.

Measuring Risk

To assess how safe something is we need to identify and measure the risks of harm associated with it. *Risk* is the probability of an adverse outcome. It may be expressed in the following terms:

- *Absolute risk* – an absolute risk must have a numerator and a denominator but it may be a proportion (e.g. 1 in 100) or a rate which includes time (e.g. 1 in 100 per year). The null value (i.e. no increased risk) is zero.
- *Relative risk* – a relative risk is a ratio and makes comparison with a specified alternative (e.g. a twofold increase compared to no treatment is a relative risk of 2). The null value is one.

Absolute risk provides more useful information than relative risk but the latter is often easier to measure. Interpreting a relative risk is difficult without knowledge of the *baseline* rate (i.e. the background probability of the effect occurring in the absence of any intervention). Several times a very small number is still a small number, whereas a small increase in the relative risk of something common could be important. This is illustrated by the comparison made in Table 2.2, showing that many more extra cases will occur in the situation where the baseline risk is high.

The fundamental problem with measuring safety is that it is much more difficult to determine that an effect is absent than to measure one that is present. We may be hoping or expecting to observe no effect but if nothing goes wrong, does that mean everything is all right?

The *rule of three* is a simple and useful tool when zero cases have been observed in a defined population (NB it cannot be used if any cases have occurred). Simply dividing the size of population by 3 approximates an upper 95% confidence limit. In practice, this is the highest value that, statistically, is reasonably likely to represent the truth. For example, if 900 patients use a new antibiotic and 0 allergic reactions occur, then it is statistically unlikely that such reactions will occur more frequently than 1 in 300 patients (i.e. 1 in 900/3).

The rule of three works very well provided the size of the population is at least 30 and thus, in the context of drug safety, it usually is applicable.

Table 2.2 Comparison between the number of extra cases produced by differing relative risks according to the level of baseline risk.

Baseline risk	Relative risk	Extra cases per million
1 in 100 (common)	1.1 (small increase)	1000
1 in 1 000 000 (very rare)	10 (large increase)	10

Safety in Practice

There are two basic components to safety:

- *Intrinsic safety* – some drugs are intrinsically and obviously safer than others at therapeutic doses. For example, the adverse reactions produced by paracetamol compared with cytotoxic drugs.
- *User-dependent safety* – the safety of a drug can also depend on how it is used. For example, monitoring white blood cell count in users of clozapine can completely prevent reduction in white blood cells to a level that would potentially have fatal consequences. Using the drug without such monitoring is therefore clearly less safe than following the recommended procedure. Another example of safety being user-dependent would be giving penicillin to someone who is allergic to it, perhaps because that information has been ignored or is not available. In such a case, the safeguard (i.e. means of minimising the risk) is avoidance of a specific drug in a particular individual. Using an appropriate dose of medicine is an example of practising risk minimisation that applies to most therapeutic situations.

The amount of safety knowledge available for a drug depends on how much it has been studied and used. Broadly, there are four categories of safety in respect of the amount of knowledge available:

1) *Well-established* – drugs that have been widely used for many (~ 20+) years for which it is unlikely that *completely unidentified* safety issues will emerge.
2) *Established* – drugs for which there is a substantial body of evidence of safety in clinical use but not enough to meet level 1.
3) *Provisional* – all newly authorised drugs until they have been used fairly extensively in ordinary practice over a period of at least 5 years. During this period such drugs are normally under *additional monitoring* (see Glossary) and their safety in ordinary practice needs to be studied proactively.
4) *Limited* – all investigational drugs and the following situations where the drug might be authorised on limited safety information:
   - Small populations eligible for treatment (e.g. rare diseases, treatments for which are known as *orphan drugs*). An example is Gaucher's disease, a lysosomal storage disorder, which is usually treated with a recombinant glucocerebrosidase.
   - Drugs with important benefits or where there is great clinical need (i.e. situations where potentially large risks might be acceptable, such as in advanced cancer).

A logical principle following from this categorisation is that *all* use of drugs in category 4 should be associated with systematic collection of safety information.

It is important to recognise that drugs in the well-established category are not necessarily safer than those in lower categories (and so on), only that more information is available about their safety.

Risk–Benefit Balance

As absolute safety is an unattainable goal, the aim is to use medicines with an *acceptable level of safety*. Various factors need to be considered in judging whether safety is or is not acceptable:

- The level of *absolute* risk(s) and the potential health consequences.
- The benefit(s) expected, also measured in absolute terms.
- The seriousness of the disease for which treatment is given.
- The risks and benefits of alternative approaches.
- The perspective and circumstances of the individual who is to be exposed.

In practice, therefore, whether safety is acceptable cannot be divorced from efficacy and expected benefits. The harms and benefits of a medicine are balanced at two levels:

1) *Population level* – this is a regulatory and research-based task and a question of whether, overall, the benefits that will accrue from availability of a medicine will exceed the expected harms.
2) *Individual level* – this is made by the clinician in consultation with the patient and takes into account factors such as the patient's previous treatment, disease severity and the patient's circumstances and preferences.

The process of balancing harms and benefits is a judgemental one and an element of judgement is always likely to remain, despite promising attempts that have been made to develop mathematical tools to aid the process at the population level. The term risk–benefit ratio has often been used but is best avoided. A ratio implies one number divided by another and even if two simple numbers were available to summarise risks and benefits, what would a ratio of, say, 1.5 mean? Conceptually it is preferable to use an additive process in *risk–benefit assessment* and the resulting balance becomes analogous to a financial balance, which is either positive or negative. Ideally, a balance sheet would be constructed and the debits (i.e. the ADRs) would be subtracted from the credits (i.e. the expected benefits), it is to be hoped leaving a positive balance. The problems are that the credits and debits are not usually measurable in the same way and there is often uncertainty about the size of some of the entries. Nevertheless, such an analogy is helpful in assessing whether to achieve these benefits it is reasonable (or not) to accept these risks of harm.

Lack of Benefit

The efficacy and effectiveness of drugs is not considered in any detail in this book because pharmacovigilance is primarily about clinical safety of medicines. However, the expected benefits of a drug are an important factor when considering whether safety is acceptable, and the overall balance of risks and benefits for at least one indication must be considered positive if a drug is to remain on the market. Conversely, when a drug is initially launched there must be evidence of efficacy and potential benefit, but this does not mean that the drug will be beneficial to all patients (many drugs do not work in surprisingly high proportions of patients) or that its 'real world' level of effectiveness will be sufficient for the risk–benefit balance to be considered positive, or remain constant over time.

The development of resistance to antibiotics is a good example of diminishing effectiveness. If there is no longer any expectation of benefit, then there can be no level of safety that will lead to a positive risk–benefit balance. At the individual level, lack of efficacy can sometimes be regarded as having serious safety implications (and therefore potentially reportable as a suspected ADR), for example if contraceptive products or devices fail, resulting in unintended pregnancies.

Causation – Was the Drug Responsible?

Deciding whether a drug is responsible for an AE is very often the most important question facing scientists working in the field of pharmacovigilance. Yet, it is rarely completely straightforward, whether the matter is being considered at the level of an individual patient or in terms of study data for various populations. As in the case of risk–benefit assessment, a judgement is often necessary and there are some principles to be applied. There are some similarities in approach between the two levels mentioned, although they are considered separately here.

Causality Assessment in Individual Cases

Many causality algorithms and categorisation systems have been proposed but none has gained universal acceptance, and the value of assessing this for each individual report of a suspected ADR has been questioned. It may be more efficient to reserve such assessment for a series of cases which might represent a new and/or important safety issue. Systematic assessment of causality in individual cases occurring in clinical trials is generally a weaker approach to assessing causality than comparison of numerical counts. However, in post-marketing surveillance, and especially in prescription-event monitoring (PEM) studies (see Chapter 3), causality assessment of individual AEs can be important in determining which may be related to the medicine and which represent background clinical events.

When individual case causality assessment is to be performed, there are usually four categories into which a case might be placed following analysis of all available clinical information:

1) *Probable* – the balance of information available supports causation. Usually, evidence of a 'positive rechallenge' (reoccurrence of the AE on readministration of the same dose of the suspect medicine) is required for this category.
2) *Possible* – some of the available information is in favour of and some against causation. For this category, usually evidence of a 'positive dechallenge' (resolution of the AE symptoms after stopping the suspect medicine) is required.
3) *Unlikely* – the balance of information available is against causation. For example, it is more likely that other factors (e.g. the patient's condition) have caused the AE.
4) *Unassessable* – a reasonable judgement cannot be made, often because key information is missing.

In making such judgements there are four broad areas to consider:

1) *Temporal relationships* – what was the time relationship between starting treatment and the onset of the event. If treatment was stopped ('dechallenge') or restarted ('rechallenge'), did the event abate and/or recur?

2) *Alternative causes* – are there concomitant diseases and other medications or non-drug exposures that could explain the event?

3) *Nature of the event* – some clinical events are often caused by drugs and immediately suggest a relationship (e.g. certain types of skin reactions such as toxic epidermal necrolysis; see Chapter 7).

4) *Plausibility* – is the reaction already recognised with this drug (or similar drugs) or can a biological mechanism be postulated based on the pharmacology of the drug?

In terms of temporal association, sometimes causation can be definitely excluded; for example, ADRs cannot start before the drug is given (although drugs can worsen existing diseases). On the other hand, a positive rechallenge in the absence of alternative causes is generally considered to be strong evidence for causation. While most ADRs start early on in treatment this is not invariably true, as reflected in the time course element of the DoTS classification already discussed.

Merely because an alternative cause can be identified does not mean that it was responsible. Possible other causes are often called 'confounding factors' and when they are present, cases are said to be 'confounded'. This is rather loose use of the word (see Figure 2.1) and best avoided.

The issues of nature of the event and plausibility need to be considered with some caution – these factors may add to the arguments for causation, but a clinical event that is not normally known to be drug-related or the absence of any information supporting plausibility is not strong evidence against it. Absence of evidence is not the same as evidence of absence.

Assessing Causality from Clinical Trial Data

One of the main reasons why data from randomised controlled trials are considered to be the gold standard is that, in principle, observed differences between randomised groups should be attributable to the different treatments (i.e. causal). Other explanations are still possible, for example differences could simply be due to chance or caused by various biases, particularly in relation to what is being measured. Problems with the randomisation may also occur – such as that it may not have been carried out properly. Sometimes, as a result of bad luck, randomisation may not have worked to produce groups that were adequately balanced at baseline in terms of important factors that may predict the outcome of interest. While all these alternative explanations need to be considered, when a difference that looks important is observed in a randomised trial, causation is the most likely explanation. If the trial has adequate statistical power (and the observed difference is statistically significant), the groups were well-balanced at baseline and the measurements are objective or blinded, then no great element of judgement is required to accept that such a difference between treatments is likely to be real.

Causality in Non-Randomised Studies – The Problems of Bias and Confounding

For study data that are not randomised, assessing causation requires much more judgement and is often a source of debate. When such studies find a difference, this is known as an *association*. In terms of chance, the issues are much the same as for randomised trials, but there are many more types of biases that may be relevant. In the real world, people tend to do things for a reason and patients who are given particular treatments may be selected according to factors that are relevant to the outcome of interest. For example, patients using coxibs (see Chapter 1) are often selected on the basis of being at higher baseline risk of gastrointestinal bleeding than patients using traditional anti-inflammatory drugs. Non-randomised comparative studies that did not address this bias would therefore be likely to (wrongly) observe the opposite of what is found in trials. A further potential bias is that losses to follow-up are more likely than in trials and the reasons why people are 'lost' from studies may not be random. For example, patients could be lost from follow-up because they have died from an ADR.

Aside from the greater problem of bias, there is also the problem of *confounding* in non-randomised studies. A confounder has a triangular relationship with an exposure (usually a drug) and outcome (AE of interest; Figure 2.1). When it is present, the risk of the outcome is affected and whether or not it is present also varies according to the exposure status. Age is a good example of a perennial confounder – in very simple terms, older people tend to use more drugs and have more adverse outcomes. Therefore there is a need to be sure that any observed association is not simply a consequence of that. A randomised study will, unless it is small, tend to balance the groups for age – or indeed any confounder – largely circumventing this problem.

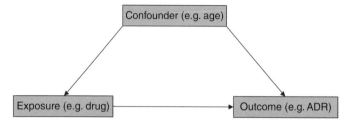

Figure 2.1 The triangular relationship between a confounder, an exposure and an outcome. By influencing both the probability of being exposed and the probability of the outcome occurring, a confounder distorts the relationship of interest (i.e. between the exposure and outcome).

In principle, confounding can be dealt with, either in the study design (e.g. by matching patients or groups so that relevant factors are balanced) or in the analysis by statistical adjustment. However, to do so requires that all potential confounders are identified and adequately measured. Smoking is another common confounder and knowledge of smoking status in terms of (say) current, ex- or non-smoker is fairly crude given that there may be a close relationship between the precise amount smoked and the risk of the outcome. The possibility that confounding has not been fully addressed is called *residual confounding* and this is often a possible alternative explanation to causation when data come from non-randomised studies.

Using the Bradford Hill Criteria to Assess Causality

When chance, bias and confounding are considered unlikely, causation is possible but still cannot be assumed as an explanation for an association based on non-randomised data. Often, there are a series of studies or various types of data that bear on this question. In this context, nine criteria first described by Bradford Hill in the 1960s are still used. Five of these can be summarised as follows:

- *Strength* – the stronger an association is, the less likely it is to be explained by other factors.
- *Consistency* – repeated observation of an association in different studies and under different conditions support causation.
- *Specificity* – a few ADRs are completely unique syndromes (some examples were given earlier) and their specificity means that causation is hardly in doubt.

- *Temporality* – exposure to the suspect medicine must precede outcomes in a consistent manner.
- *Biological gradient* – is there evidence of dose- or duration-related risk?

The final four criteria are *plausibility, coherence, supportive experimental evidence* and *analogy*. These are related by a theme of whether the association fits with existing scientific knowledge and beliefs. If so, then causation is more likely but newly identified associations may not fit, so absence of any (or all) of these criteria does not preclude an association being causal.

In general terms, the more criteria that are met, the more likely an association is to be causal. However, there is no simple formula for adding up these criteria and coming to a definitive answer. Professional judgement is required for such assessments and Bradford Hill's criteria are merely a conceptual framework for making such a judgement. It is worth noting that some of the criteria (e.g. temporality, dose–response, plausibility) are analogous to what was described for the assessment of causality in individual cases.

Conclusions

This chapter has considered the most fundamental concepts in pharmacovigilance: what is an adverse effect of a medicine, how do we know that it really is an adverse reaction, what is safety and on what basis do we consider a treatment to be safe? We have discussed the concept of measuring risk and the differences between relative and absolute risk. The concept of the balance of risk and benefit is important because a key goal of the pharmacovigilance process is to ensure that the risks of drug treatments are outweighed by the benefits. Finally, we have covered the concepts behind causality assessment, a basic and vital tool in pharmacovigilance practice. The next step is to consider in more detail the various kinds of data that help us to answer such questions in relation to specific medicines and safety issues.

3

Types and Sources of Data

The safety of medicines is under evaluation throughout the drug development cycle. This process starts before humans are exposed, and continues during the clinical development and post-marketing phases. Broadly, the safety of a medicine is tested in four phases, each of which produces different types of data:

1) Pre-clinical (animal) studies
2) Healthy human volunteer studies (Phase I)
3) Clinical trials (Phases II and III)
4) Post-marketing surveillance (Phase IV)

Although there is a natural sequence defined by the above order, the phases are not entirely distinct. Sometimes, new pre-clinical studies are undertaken for authorised products and, as we saw in Chapter 1, clinical trials are increasingly becoming important post-marketing. Systematic reviews and meta-analysis are important tools for bringing together data from multiple studies. Although they have usually been applied in the assessment of efficacy, their use for safety purposes is increasing.

Pre-clinical Studies

Pre-clinical studies are usually conducted in rodents (rabbit, mouse, rat) and dogs or primates (monkeys). They aim to establish dosage levels below which toxicity is not observed and to identify the organs

An Introduction to Pharmacovigilance, Second Edition. Patrick Waller and Mira Harrison-Woolrych.
© 2017 John Wiley & Sons Ltd. Published 2017 by John Wiley & Sons Ltd.

adversely affected by higher doses. The most important potential effects studied are:

- Major organ toxicity
- Acute and chronic toxicity
- Carcinogenicity
- Mutagenicity (i.e. able to induce genetic mutation)
- Teratogenicity (i.e. producing physical defects in the embryo).

Even at this stage, some adverse effects might be acceptable, depending on the ultimate target population for the drug. For example, adverse reproductive effects could be considered less important for a drug that is to be used exclusively in an elderly population.

Adverse drug reactions (ADRs) may not be specific to particular species. When studies in animals demonstrate major toxicity, further drug development is usually precluded and the level of toxicity in humans remains unknown. When no major toxicity has been demonstrated in animals, development can proceed into humans but some ADRs appear to be specific to humans (e.g. the multi-system oculomucocutaneous syndrome caused by the beta-blocker practolol). It is generally accepted that thalidomide teratogenicity was not predictable from animal studies.

Generally, the predictive value of pre-clinical studies for human toxicity is not more than moderate and discussions continue about the relevance of these studies to human use. Overall, they provide only limited reassurance that use in humans will be acceptably safe.

Human Volunteer Studies (Phase I)

For most medicines, the first human exposure takes place in healthy volunteers but cytotoxic drugs used to treat cancers are an exception. Participants are very closely monitored with clinical supervision and resuscitation equipment must be immediately to hand. The purposes are to establish a possible dosage regimen, investigate how the drug is handled by the body and what the effects are on a variety of standard parameters (e.g. pulse and blood pressure, ECG, haematology). Assuming the drug appears to have no major untoward effects, it can then be studied in clinical trials that include patients with the target disease(s).

Healthy volunteer (or Phase I) studies have generally had a good safety record over a long period of time but, occasionally, major adverse reactions do occur. In 2006, all six of the first humans treated with the monoclonal antibody TGN1412 in London rapidly developed multi-organ failure. The incident was investigated in detail by the UK regulatory authority who concluded that the reactions were an unexpected biological effect. A further unexpected and serious incident occurred in France in 2016 when administration of escalating doses of BIA 10-2474, a fatty acid amide hydrolase inhibitor, to healthy volunteers led to one death and three cases of serious neurological damage in healthy volunteers. In that instance, about 80 people had previously been given the drug without similar effects being observed.

Clinical Trials (Phase II and III Studies)

Clinical trials are usually designed to study both efficacy and safety, but efficacy is usually the primary end-point. The design of such trials incorporates various features to minimise bias such as randomisation to treatment groups, blinding of subjects and observers/investigators to treatment allocation, and validated measurement instruments. Initially, fairly small Phase II trials are conducted; these tend to be focused on efficacy and dosage requirements. Larger Phase III trials are then conducted and form the key element of the safety database prior to marketing. All adverse events occurring in patients after exposure to the drug and a comparator (which can be a placebo or an alternative active drug) are systematically recorded. In order to minimise measurement bias, it is usual to 'blind' all study participants (i.e. patients and clinicians, which is known as 'double blinding') to the treatments given or, if that is not possible, to 'blind' those who are involved in assessing the outcomes (a form of 'single blinding'), particularly if there is any subjectivity involved.

In clinical trials, the data are analysed to identify adverse events that occur at significantly higher rates on the medicinal product of interest than on comparators. Usually, the data from all pre-licensing trials are pooled in a global safety analysis for presentation to regulatory authorities. Clinical trials will identify most common adverse reactions but often have important limitations, including:

- Selection of patients – those at greatest risk of ADRs, or those who have not responded to similar medicines, are often excluded.
- Study size – the numbers of patients studied is generally not enough to identify rare but serious ADRs.

- The artificial conditions – patients are likely to be more closely monitored than in real life.
- Measurement of surrogate markers of effect rather than 'hard' end-points.
- The duration of follow-up is usually short, weeks or months rather than years.

At the conclusion of a clinical trial, patients may be continued on the treatment and followed-up for a period of months or years, generating more long-term safety experience. These are known as 'open-label' extensions as it known which treatment is being taken. When clinical trials are conducted entirely after marketing, they may provide important new safety information, provided that they contain enough patients, have few exclusion criteria and clinically relevant outcomes that are easily measured (e.g. mortality). Such studies are often called 'large simple trials'.

During the clinical trial phase of drug development, there is a major safety focus on the protection of trial participants. Investigators are obliged to document and report serious adverse events promptly. If a serious and unexpected suspected adverse reaction (SUSAR; see Chapter 5) occurs, then the case should be unblinded and reported to regulatory authorities. The identification of a serious new hazard may lead to a trial – or even the whole development programme – being stopped. In all clinical trials there should be safety monitoring arrangements in place (including a data monitoring committee) to oversee unblinded safety results as they emerge, possibly in accordance with a pre-planned series of sequential analyses. Care needs to be taken so that such procedures do not compromise the integrity of the trial, but the need to ensure that trial participants are not exposed to unnecessary risk is paramount. In this respect there is an ethical dimension to safety in trials, and in most countries clinical studies require ethics committee approval before commencement. Ethical issues are considered further in Chapter 8.

Post-marketing Surveillance (Phase IV Studies)

Because of the limitations of pre-marketing studies, safety can only be regarded as provisional when a new medicine is first marketed. There is a need to collect more evidence arising from 'real world' usage, which differs from use of the medicine in a clinical trial in several important ways, including larger and different populations exposed and less formal monitoring. Spontaneous ADR reporting is generally regarded as the cornerstone of such monitoring and its main purpose is for the detection of 'signals' of previously unrecognised hazards (see Chapter 4): hypothesis generation. Formal pharmacoepidemiological studies should then be designed to investigate and characterise serious possible ADRs: hypothesis testing.

The extent to which the safety of a new drug can be studied post-marketing depends considerably on how much it is used. If uptake is slow, then it may be some time before there is sufficient exposure to conduct a formal study. On the other hand, if uptake is rapid, then many people may suffer the consequences of an important safety problem while it is being identified and investigated.

Spontaneous ADR Reporting Systems

The primary purpose of spontaneous ADR reporting is to provide early warnings or 'signals' of previously unrecognised drug toxicity. As discussed in Chapter 1, the method was developed in the 1960s in response to the thalidomide tragedy and is now well-established throughout the developed world and in some developing countries. Health professionals are the key original source of spontaneous reports, but in recent years patient reporting has become widely accepted, although its value in signal detection is not fully established. In recent years, electronic transmission of all reports has become the norm between pharmaceutical companies and regulatory authorities in most countries and is progressing in terms of initial transmission from health professionals in many parts of the world.

Spontaneous ADR reporting can be defined as a scheme for collating individual case reports of suspected ADRs, operated for the primary purpose of detecting unknown, potentially seriously harmful effects of drugs. As discussed in Chapter 2, individual cases can be assessed for causation using established principles. However, except in the very rare circumstance whereby a drug causes a previously unidentified syndrome (i.e. an apparently completely specific drug–event association), a series of spontaneous ADR reports provides only limited evidence of causation. Generally therefore, data from these schemes raise questions rather than provide answers.

Today, many spontaneous ADR reporting systems are in operation around the world and these are generally effective, but they are not a panacea for two main reasons. First, the output is essentially only a 'signal', which is a possible association requiring further evaluation and investigation and some signals will inevitably turn out to be false positives (i.e. not related to the drug). Secondly, the method is far from perfect in rapidly detecting all unrecognised ADRs. There will also be false negatives, which are ultimately detected by other methods, e.g. practolol and oculo-mucocutaneous syndrome, as discussed in Chapter 1).

Key Elements of Spontaneous Reporting Programmes

Spontaneous ADR reporting is conceptually simple. Reports are submitted on a voluntary basis and information is entered on to a database which is screened regularly for signals. The main elements of a scheme which are essential to its success can be summarised as in the following sections.

Health Professionals who are Willing to Participate

The value of a spontaneous report mainly derives from the suspicion of a reporter that a drug may have been responsible for a particular event. Most national programmes now encourage reports from any health professional involved in the patient's care including doctors, pharmacists, nurses and midwives. When a report is submitted by a patient or carer (or a health professional who is not the patient's usual carer), there is much to be gained by follow-up with the patient's regular doctor (general practitioners in many countries) who usually has the most clinical information about the patient concerned.

Cooperation from clinicians is essential for successful spontaneous reporting schemes and, in practice in most countries, reporting is invariably voluntary. Although some countries have 'mandatory' ADR reporting schemes for health professionals, they do not always have markedly higher reporting rates per head of the population, because usually there is no practical mechanism of enforcement. The reasons why some health professionals are prepared to report (and why some countries have much higher rates of reporting) are not fully under-stood and are likely to be multifactorial, including other elements of reporting schemes.

Simplicity in Submission of Reports

If busy health professionals are to submit reports voluntarily, they are only likely to do so if the process is straightforward. Reporting needs to be facilitated by the ready availability of clearly laid out forms which are simple to complete, and internationally agreed standard forms are in wide use. Both paper and electronic forms need to be made available, the former with free postage.

Electronic reporting methods are increasingly important and several national pharmacovigilance centres have now developed apps for phones and other devices. Most centres will accept reports in different forms, including verbally (e.g. by telephone), handwritten (hard copy form) or electronic submission. However, with all methods, an individual case report form should be completed.

Prompt Entry of Reports on to a Database

It is important to ensure prompt data entry of reports on to databases to avoid backlogs and to ensure that reports containing vital new information are assessed as soon as possible. Most national schemes have standard operating procedures to ensure timely data entry and evaluation of reports.

Data entry involves coding both the suspect medicine (and concomitant medicines) and the suspected ADR. Standard dictionaries should be used for coding. A drugs dictionary is required for coding medicines and the most commonly used is the one maintained by the World Health Organization (WHO). This uses the Anatomical Therapeutic Chemical (ATC) classification system and contains around 50 000 drugs.

Coding and Assessment of ADR Reports

For coding ADRs, international medical terminology dictionaries are used, in particular the Medical Dictionary for Regulatory Activities (MedDRA) or the WHO Adverse Reaction Terminology (WHO-ART). Other details from the report, for example, patient details (age, sex, etc.), time to onset of the ADR, severity of the reaction and the outcome for the patient, should also be entered into the database. Whether a full causality assessment is done for each report (see Chapter 4) varies from country to country, as does the degree of clinical assessment of individual reports.

Follow-up of Reports

Reporters may be contacted for follow-up (i.e. provision of additional detailed clinical information, e.g. results of investigations, autopsy reports) or ascertainment of the outcome subsequent to initial submission. In most schemes, follow-up is selective, dependent on the perceived importance of a report and the extent to which information important for its evaluation has already been provided. In some schemes, all reporters are contacted after assessment of the initial report, with further information requested as required. A simple principle is that all serious reports should be followed-up.

Analytical Tools to Detect Signals

Analytical methods are now used in many schemes to detect to signals from spontaneously reported ADRs and these are discussed in detail in Chapter 4.

Processes for Dealing with Signals

Once a signal has been identified, the next step is to evaluate all the relevant available information, including that derived from other data sources. Because signal evaluation is resource-intensive and large numbers of signals can be detected in some databases, interim steps have been proposed to prioritise them including triage and impact analysis. These tools and the principles of signal evaluation are discussed in Chapter 4.

Feedback to Reporters

In order to complete a feedback loop, information must also flow back to reporters through acknowledgement, provision of data and bulletins describing evaluated signals. Methods of feedback to reporters vary among national centres, but electronic methods are increasingly important.

Recent Spontaneous Reporting Data from the UK Yellow Card Scheme

To illustrate the nature of the data received through spontaneous ADR reporting in a developed country, we assessed information from the Medicines and Healthcare products Regulatory Agency (MHRA) in the UK. In this country, which has a population of around 60 million, the total number of spontaneously reported ADRs has increased in recent years. In 2015, a total of 39 046 reports were received compared to 21 419 in 2006. During this period the proportions of reports received from different sources did not vary greatly. Overall, the proportion received from healthcare professionals was 46%, with 40% being received via the pharmaceutical industry and 14% from patients or their carers. The proportions of reports that were fatal (5%), serious (79%) and non-serious (16%) were also quite stable.

During the period 2011–2015 more than 1000 reports per year were received in every 10-year age band up to the age of 90. One of the main age-related changes in this period has been an increase in children aged 0–10 years, in whom the number of reports has roughly doubled. During 2011–2015, the system organ classes most commonly used to classify the reported reactions have consistently been general disorders (a category used to cover reactions that do not clearly fit into a specific organ system, e.g. malaise), neurological disorders, gastrointestinal and skin disorders. These data only illustrate what has been reported and may be subject to various biases. For example, it is unlikely that the true frequency of ADRs in young children has increased and the trend in the data is much more likely to represent an effect of steps taken to promote awareness and reporting of ADRs in children.

Spontaneous Reporting Around the World

Spontaneous reporting schemes are well-established throughout the developed world and have also been set up in many developing countries. Most national schemes are run by the medicines regulatory agency but other models exist, for example in the Netherlands and in New Zealand, where the monitoring centre is a separate institution. Some larger countries have regional centres which may serve as a local base for the submission, handling and follow-up of reports, and/or assist in promoting reporting and education about ADRs. In France, the whole country is covered by such regional centres with a coordinating group based at the French medicines agency. In the UK, only part of the country is covered by regional centres and in other areas reports are submitted and handled centrally.

In most countries, pharmaceutical companies have legal obligations to submit spontaneous adverse reaction reports (see Chapter 5) and these are entered on to the national database. There is some variation among countries as to the proportion of reports that come via the industry (e.g. a large majority do so in Germany, the USA and

Singapore, but the proportion is less in the UK). There is a potential for duplication of reports which a clinician submits to both industry and agency and also because more than one clinician can report the same case. A systematic approach to screening databases for duplicates is required and this task has become more difficult as confidentiality restrictions have increased.

International standards for ADR reporting have been developed since the late 1980s through the Council for International Organizations of Medical Sciences (CIOMS) and International Council on Harmonisation (ICH) (see Chapter 6).

Strengths and Weaknesses of Spontaneous Reporting

The main strengths of spontaneous reporting lie in its simplicity, that it can be universally applied (all drugs, all the time) and in its ability to rapidly capture clinical suspicions that may otherwise to go unrecorded. In theory, spontaneous reporting is cheap to run, although globally much resource is now put into it and, overall, it is not as efficient as it could be because of duplicated efforts.

The main limitations of the method are inevitable and unquantifiable under-reporting, and the potential for the data to be misunderstood. Curiously, most of the biases affecting the data are actually positive features, which reflect the way these schemes are promoted. Thus, a report is more likely to be submitted if the ADR is serious, unrecognised or relates to a new drug – all features that are desirable. The other major bias – the effect of publicity – is often undesirable but can only occur once a hazard has been recognised by some means. It therefore does not detract from the primary purpose of the method, but it does mean that interpretation of the data during subsequent monitoring is fraught with difficulty.

Misperceptions of the data are common. For example, the information that (say) 50 fatal suspected ADRs have been reported with a particular drug sounds worrying, particularly to lay people. However, this cannot be interpreted without considering carefully several factors, including the nature of the possible ADRs, what the drug is used for, how much it has been used and what other evidence might be available to support a causal link. Spontaneous ADR databases contain a fair amount of background 'noise', in that suspected reactions were not actually caused by the drug, but this point is often not appreciated and may lead to misinterpretation of these types of data.

It is important to recognise that spontaneous ADR reporting is most likely to detect signals of relatively rare ADRs when the background incidence of the disease is low. Relatively common ADRs are likely to have been detected earlier in drug development by clinical trials and detecting rare ADRs is difficult when the background incidence of the event is high. This is because clinicians are not surprised to see cases of common diseases (such as myocardial infarction).

Although spontaneous ADR reporting is a well-established method, both the utility of the schemes and the data they generate are frequently subject to misperceptions. For example, a report prepared by politicians in 2005 described the UK scheme as 'widely considered to be failing', an assessment that no scientist experienced in the field would accept. One of the main reasons for this assessment seemed to be the problem of under-reporting, but this is inherent in the method. There seem to be some widely held myths about under-reporting which can be questioned. The first is that the overall degree of under-reporting approximates to 90% (i.e. only 10% of ADRs are reported). The evidence base for this is very limited and the reality is that the degree of under-reporting varies considerably in relation to factors such as seriousness, the novelty of the drug and the nature of the suspected ADR. Critics also believe that the effectiveness of these schemes might be directly proportional to the number of reports received and that under-reporting undermines the whole concept. These perceptions are not based on hard evidence and do not reflect decades of experience with the method.

Despite the limitations discussed, it is clear that we will continue to need systems that fulfil the purpose of spontaneous ADR reporting schemes for the foreseeable future. It is also clear that, for most drugs, relying on spontaneous reporting alone is insufficient and a proactive approach to studying safety using pharmacoepidemiological studies is required.

Pharmacoepidemiological Studies

Pharmacoepidemiology is the scientific discipline of studying drug effects in populations, which is largely focused on measuring potential harms and safety in the post-marketing phase. Pharmacoepidemiological studies are *observational* (whereas clinical trials are *experimental* or *interventional*) – they attempt to measure effects under real-life conditions. Larger populations can be studied than in clinical trials and the findings are likely to be generally applicable. However, as discussed in Chapter 2, without randomisation, attribution of causation is more difficult. Observational studies provide evidence of association (or no association) and a judgement then has to be made on causation taking into account all the available information. To recap from Chapter 2, four possible explanations for a positive association generally have to be considered:

1) *Chance* – taking into account the level of statistical significance
2) *Bias* – a systematic error
3) *Confounding* – the association is produced by a third factor which is related to both drug use and outcome
4) *Causal effect* – the other explanations can reasonably be excluded, as assessed by Bradford Hill's criteria.

There are two principal types of study design:

• *Cohort study* – all users of a medicinal product (the exposure) are identified and followed-up to determine what events or ADRs occur (the outcomes).

• *Case–control study* – all cases of the disease (the outcome), the putative reactions are identified and their use of the drugs of interest (the exposures) are compared with controls without this disease.

A case–control study may be *nested* within a cohort study (i.e. cases and controls are all drawn from a clearly defined cohort). This is an efficient design which is commonly used in pharmacoepidemiology.

Attempts are made in the design and analysis of pharmacoepidemiology studies to minimise possible biases, and to identify and adjust for confounding factors. Typically, a cohort study will measure both absolute and relative risks, whereas a case–control study will usually only measure odds ratios which generally approximate to relative risks. In both cases the data may be summarised in two-by-two tables, as shown in Tables 3.1 and 3.2.

Note that the starting point in Table 3.1 is two cohorts of 10 000 subjects who are followed-up and that relatively few of them (as is usually the case) experience the outcome of interest. The key estimate from this study is the attributable risk of 0.3%, which means that about 1 patient in 333 (i.e. the inverse of 0.3%) will experience the event because of the drug, if the association is causal. The relative risk of 2.5 means that two

Table 3.1 Example of risk data from a cohort study design.

	Used drug	No drug	Totals
Event	50 (a)	20 (b)	70
No event	9950 (c)	9980 (d)	19 930
Totals	10 000 (a + c)	10 000 (b + d)	20 000

Risk of event on drug: a/(a + c) or 50/10 000 = 0.5%.
Risk of event in comparison group: b/(b + d) or 20/10 000 = 0.2%.
Absolute risk attributable to drug: [a/(a + c)] − [b/(b + d)] or 0.5% minus 0.2% = 0.3%.
Relative risk: [a/(a + c)]/[b/(b + d)] or 0.5%/0.2% = 2.5.

Table 3.2 Example of risk data from a case–control study design.

	Cases	Controls	Totals
Used drug	10 (a)	20 (b)	30
No drug	90 (c)	480 (d)	570
Totals	100	500	600

Odds ratio (approximate relative risk) = ad/bc = 4800/1800 = 2.67.

and half times as many drug-treated patients experienced the event in comparison with those who did not receive the drug.

Note that the starting point in Table 3.2 is a series of identified cases of the outcome of interest. Prior exposure to the drug is then evaluated, but only a few of the cases had used the drug. It is usual to include more controls because they are easier to find and this will increase the statistical power of the study. Proportionately fewer controls had used the drug and therefore the odds ratio in this study was more than two. As the odds ratio approximates to a relative risk, these two studies give a similar answer but, as discussed in Chapter 2, the additional information provided by the cohort study that the absolute risk is 0.3% is very useful. This cannot be calculated in a standard case–control study.

Pharmacoepidemiological studies can be set up from scratch ('field' studies) but large studies are now almost invariably conducted by using data collected for other purposes, such as from the Clinical Practice Research Datalink in the UK or various health maintenance/insurance organisations in the USA.

In order to be useful for pharmacoepidemiological purposes, a database must provide:

- Prescription records
- Adverse event data
- Demographic and other health information.

Studies can be carried out solely using information on a database, particularly if the quality of the data has been validated. However, it is considered good practice to seek additional information from clinical records, particularly to confirm that there is adequate evidence to support diagnosis of the adverse event in individual cases. This can lead to some potential cases being excluded and exclusions may be specified for other reasons but, in general, these should be kept to a minimum in order to retain the advantage that such data have in representing real life.

Prescription-Event Monitoring

Prescription-event monitoring (PEM) – sometimes known as cohort event monitoring – is a pharmacoepidemiological system which was developed in New Zealand in the late 1970s and in England around 1980. The method has also proved to be valuable in Japan. It is mostly focused on new medicines, particularly those used for chronic diseases, and is complementary to spontaneous reporting as a method of identifying unexpected ADRs. In New Zealand, the Intensive Medicines Monitoring Programme (IMMP) identified many new signals during its years of operation (1977–2013).

PEM has the advantage that the number of users of the drug (i.e. the denominator population) is known and therefore that event frequencies can be quantified. An important point about the method is that all *events* are recorded (in the numerator), whether or not there is suspicion that they were drug-induced. PEM can therefore identify effects that clinicians do not recognise as being ADRs. This type of study can be used to investigate potential safety issues that have been identified during development, for example to determine the frequency of a specific ADR in real-life use or to investigate risk factors for ADRs. A further use of PEM is to perform drug utilisation studies and these include investigation of safety issues, such as the reasons patients had for stopping a medicine.

In PEM, patients taking specific medicines are identified through prescriptions written by general practitioners (GPs) and dispensed by pharmacists. In UK PEM, undertaken by the Drug Safety Research Unit (DSRU), prescription records are obtained from a central database, whereas in New Zealand PEM, prescription records are sent directly from pharmacies to the IMMP. Both methods result in the formation of nationwide cohorts of patients and using dispensing records rather than prescription records (as is the case in general practice database studies) gives a more accurate estimate of the cohort using a medicine, because up to 25% of prescriptions are never dispensed. The usual size of the cohort in PEM is about 10000 patients – almost an order of magnitude greater than the usual number studied in clinical trials before marketing.

Adverse events that occur during the monitoring period are then captured on forms/questionnaires which are sent to and completed by the patient's GP. Follow-up questionnaires can also request other information about the patient, for example clinical details which help identify risk factors for adverse events. Over many years, both the UK DSRU and the New Zealand IMMP modified PEM to conduct numerous pharmacoepidemiology studies and examine specific clinical issues. For example, an IMMP study of atypical antipsychotic medicines showed that one in five adult patients taking clozapine developed nocturnal bed-wetting.

PEM has been shown to be a useful and adaptable method to perform post-marketing safety studies. Like spontaneous reporting, PEM schemes are voluntary and in both New Zealand and the UK they have received excellent cooperation from GPs, pharmacists, other health professionals and patients. When a medicine has been studied by PEM and no important new ADRs have been identified, the data provide some reassurance about its safety. However, PEM studies are usually not large enough to identify very rare ADRs and longer term ADRs can still arise after the period of monitoring. PEM continues in the UK, but in New Zealand the IMMP was closed in 2013 because of insufficient funding.

Registries

A registry is used to collect individual patient data which can be used for epidemiological studies. Ideally, it will provide complete capture of a subpopulation based on a disease, treatment, specific exposure or outcome.

Registries are particularly useful for studying long-term effects, rare diseases and rare exposures. With regard to drug safety, some examples of registries are as follows.

Disease/outcome-based registries:

- Cancer
- Orphan diseases
- Fetal/neonatal outcomes (from pregnancy registries or birth registers).

Drug-based registries:

- As part of a risk minimisation programme (e.g. clozapine monitoring schemes)
- Drugs used to treat orphan diseases
- Medicines taken in pregnancy.

A registry that has been used to collect data on biological therapies for rheumatoid arthritis is an example of one that is based on both disease and drugs. Registries that are disease-based offer greater flexibility in terms of study design – patients not exposed to particular drugs are useful for comparative purposes.

Systematic Reviews and Meta-analysis

These are important tools in evidence-based medicine and their underlying purpose is often to guide health and treatment policies, and determine the future research agenda.

A systematic review brings together and evaluates all the relevant research relating to a particular question. Usually, such reviews focus on identifying research papers published in the scientific literature, but authors of extensive systematic reviews can also approach researchers for unpublished evidence. A group known as the Cochrane Collaboration was formed for the purpose of appraising medical treatments. Its findings are published in the Cochrane Library which is widely available, freely in some countries. Most of the focus has been on evidence of efficacy from randomised trials, but many Cochrane reviews include information on safety outcomes and an adverse event methods group has also been formed.

A meta-analysis brings together data from different studies in a quantitative way so as to provide a single overall estimate of a specified effect. When doing this, it is best to use only evidence of one particular type (e.g. from randomised trials) and the outcome(s) must be expressed in the same terms for all the studies. While meta-analysis has most often been focused on efficacy, it can be used for adverse outcomes and the method is useful for contributing to drug safety issues and risk–benefit assessments. Meta-analysis of data from observational studies is possible, but is more controversial than that from randomised controlled trials.

A meta-analysis is, in effect, a study of studies and should be conducted according to a defined protocol. As far as possible, all the relevant evidence should be included, whether published or not, but duplication has to be avoided. In the presentation of data, the individual study findings ought to be demonstrated in addition to the overall effect. Meta-analysis is not the same as simple pooling of data from several studies. Rather than merely pooling the numerators and denominators, a meta-analysis combines the observed *differences* between treatments for each study and weighs them according to the precision of the studies, so that the larger studies carry more weight.

As well as providing a combined estimate, a meta-analysis should aid understanding of the strengths and limitations of the available evidence. It is important to consider the reasons why the individual studies appear to differ in their findings. If there is a large degree of heterogeneity in the data, it is still possible to display that graphically but it may not be sensible to calculate a single overall estimate.

Conclusions

This chapter has considered the main types of data that are used in pharmacovigilance, including preclinical studies, clinical trials, spontaneous ADR data, pharmacoepidemiological studies (including case–control, cohort and PEM studies), registries, systematic reviews and meta-analysis. In summarising all these potential data sources, we have discussed their strengths and limitations. In the next chapter, we try to illustrate how such data fit into the overall process of pharmacovigilance.

4

The Process of Pharmacovigilance

Overview – A Risk Management Process

As indicated in Chapter 1, pharmacovigilance is essentially a risk management process for medicines. The process starts with identification of a possible hazard, which is then evaluated and investigated and, if necessary, some action is then taken with a view to minimising risks. Implementation requires tools for communicating with prescribers and users and the final step should be an assessment of the effectiveness of this process. The whole process of risk management is iterative because new evidence may emerge, or the measures taken may turn out to be insufficient. Rarely can a drug safety issue be considered completely and permanently resolved.

The start of the process is usually a 'signal' (something that needs to be looked at further), which may not turn out to be a true hazard. Before that can happen, there is a need to identify the signal.

Signal Detection

What is a Signal?

The World Health Organization (WHO) has defined a signal as:

> Reported information on a possible causal relationship between an adverse event and a drug, the relationship being unknown or incompletely documented previously. Usually more than a single report is required to generate a signal, depending upon the seriousness of the event and the quality of the information.

An Introduction to Pharmacovigilance, Second Edition. Patrick Waller and Mira Harrison-Woolrych.
© 2017 John Wiley & Sons Ltd. Published 2017 by John Wiley & Sons Ltd.

This definition seems mainly focused on spontaneous ADR reporting data. A broader approach would be to consider a signal as simply an alert from *any* available data source that a drug *may* be associated with a previously unrecognised hazard or that a known hazard *may* be quantitatively (e.g. more frequent) or qualitatively (e.g. more serious) different from existing knowledge. This approach is in line with the Council for International Organizations of Medical Sciences (CIOMS) VIII report (see Chapter 6), which defines a signal as:

> Information that arises from one or multiple sources (including observations and experiments), which suggests a new potentially causal association, or a new aspect of a known association, between an intervention and an event or a set of related events, either adverse or beneficial, that is judged to be of sufficient likelihood to justify verificatory action.

In practice, most signals will relate to previously unrecognised hazards, but a striking example of a signal that a known hazard was more serious than previously thought occurred in the mid-1990s. The non-steroidal anti-inflammatory drug, tiaprofenic acid, had been known to cause cystitis for over a decade, but a series of cases was then reported indicating that, if the reaction was not recognised and the drug was continued in the long term, severe chronic cystitis might occur. The outcome was that surgical resection of the bladder was often necessary, leading to permanent disability.

While some signals may be detected passively (e.g. from the medical literature), the process of signal detection should be fundamentally an active one. In terms of finding signals in large databases, it has been suggested that this is akin to looking for a needle in a haystack, although there are likely to be lots of needles to find. The term *data mining* (actively searching for patterns in large datasets) is now widely used in this context, particularly in relation to systematic detection of signals from large spontaneous ADR databases.

Processes for Signal Detection

In the context of spontaneous ADR reporting, a signal is normally a series of cases of similar suspected ADRs reported in relation to a particular medicinal product. When the suspected ADR is a condition that is rare in the general population (e.g. aplastic anaemia, toxic epidermal necrolysis), a very small number of cases associated with a single drug is unlikely to be a chance phenomenon, even if the drug has been used quite widely. Except for certain types of event that are particularly important and likely to be drug related (e.g. anaphylaxis), a single case is not usually sufficient to raise a signal. Three cases are generally considered to be the minimum number of cases needed.

The amount of drug usage (i.e. some drug exposure data) is helpful in providing context to a series of reported cases, but it is not usually critical in determining whether there is a signal that needs to be evaluated. The strength of evidence for the individual cases will be important to consider later but, initially, the key issue is whether there is an unexpectedly large enough number of cases.

In the past, various methods have been used to detect signals using spontaneous reporting data. Calculating reporting rates based on usage denominator data, as prescriptions dispensed or defined daily doses (or less accurately from estimated sales figures), may enable a signal of a particular ADR to be derived by comparison with alternative treatments. As spontaneous ADR reporting schemes are subject to a variable and unknown degree of under-reporting and denominator data derived from sales data can be very inaccurate, such comparisons are crude. They may also be biased, particularly if the drugs being compared have been marketed for different indications or durations, or if there has been significant publicity about the adverse effects of one of the drugs.

Disproportionality Approaches or Signal Detection

The other principal approach that has been for making comparisons between drugs is to use the proportions of all ADRs for a particular drug that are of a specific type – perhaps within an organ system class of reactions (e.g. gastrointestinal or cutaneous). This is known as *profiling*, a method that has an advantage over reporting rates in that it is independent of the level of usage. The data can be displayed graphically as 'ADR profiles'. This proportionate approach forms the basis of statistical methods which have been developed since the mid-1990s and are now widely used. One important advantage of these methods is that no external data (e.g. usage) are required – they are entirely based on information present on a single database.

The basic concept behind such measures of 'disproportionality' is whether more reports have been received for a particular drug–reaction combination than might have been expected as background noise. When all drugs are considered together, large ADR databases tend to have fairly stable proportions of particular reactions over time. That proportion is used as a baseline for comparison –to determine what would be expected if there was no signal. For example, in the UK Yellow Card database in the mid-1990s, there were nearly 600 000 suspected reactions which had been reported to any drug over a period of 30 years. Almost 800 of these (about 0.13%) were classified as 'uveitis' (inflammation of the middle layer of the eye). A few years earlier, a new anti-tuberculous drug,rifabutin, had been introduced and some 41 cases of uveitis were reported as suspected ADRs to this drug. In total, only 55 reactions of any kind had been reported with rifabutin by that time (i.e. 75% of them were uveitis). In this example, the expected proportion of uveitis reports (derived from placing all other drugs together) was 0.13% but the observed value for rifabutin was 75%. Dividing 75/0.13 yields a number well over 500 – this is known as the *proportional reporting ratio (PRR)*. The 'null value' of a PRR is 1 and the calculation is made from a two-by-two table, as shown in Table 4.1.

As can be seen from the statistical tests, this was very unlikely to have occurred by chance and is a very extreme finding. In fact, this signal was quite obvious without using mathematics. The approach is more likely to be useful in identifying signals that might otherwise be missed when the PRR is much lower – say in the range of 1–10. In general, experience has shown that a PRR of 3 or more represents a degree of disproportionality worth looking into further, providing it is

Table 4.1 Example of proportional reporting ratio (PRR) calculation: rifabutin and uveitis.

	Rifabutin	All other drugs	Totals
Uveitis	41	754	795
All other ADRs	14	591 958	591 972
Totals	55	592 712	592 767

Proportion of ADRs that are uveitis with rifabutin = 41/55 (i.e. 0.75).
Proportion of ADRs that are uveitis for all drugs 754/592 712 = 0.0013.
PRR = 0.75/0.0013 = 556.
Chi-squared (1 degree of freedom) = 22 000, $P \ll 0.00001$.

unlikely to have occurred by chance, that is, the value of chi-squared exceeds 4 (roughly the 5% level of statistical significance).

Going back to the point about generally needing three cases, it is therefore possible to regard the following as cut-off points for a minimum signal:

- PRR >3
- Chi-squared >4
- N = 3 or more.

Using such criteria, whole databases can be screened regularly by calculating two-by-two tables for all drug–reaction combinations to identify those that most need further attention.

A useful way of visualising the data is to plot, on logarithmic scales, the PRR against the value of chi-squared using the number of reports (N) as the symbol (Figure 4.1). The vertical and horizontal lines represent the cut-off points and everything in the upper right-hand quadrant is a signal of an unexpected degree of disproportionality. Note that the 41 cases of uveitis reported with rifabutin appear in this quadrant as one of the most extreme data points.

Another useful way of looking at the data is to plot the PRR over time (Figure 4.2). In the historical example given in Figure 4.2, the angiotensin converting enzyme (ACE) inhibitor captopril was first marketed in 1982 but it took until 1986 before cough was recognised

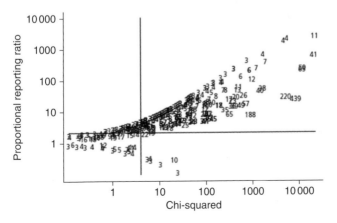

Figure 4.1 Plot of proportional reporting ratio (PRR) vs. chi-squared (from UK spontaneous ADR reporting data); the number of reports is used as the symbol.

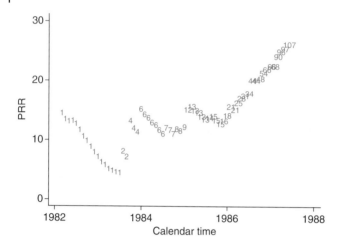

Figure 4.2 Plot of PRR over time for captopril and cough (from UK spontaneous ADR reporting data); the number of reports is used as the symbol.

as an adverse reaction with this class of drug. Like thalidomide and practolol, the first indication of this association appeared in the published medical literature. By the beginning of 1986 there were at least 15 reports in the UK ADR database and the criteria discussed earlier would have been met some 2 years earlier when there were four reports and a PRR above 10. Note how the PRR fluctuates over time – ADR databases are dynamic – and that the increase in the period 1986–1988 is most likely to have been an effect of publicity about the reaction.

The PRR is just one of several measures of disproportionality that have been used. A reporting odds ratio (ROR) can be calculated from the same two-by-two table and has been mostly used in the Netherlands. The WHO Uppsala Monitoring Centre (UMC) uses the information component (IC) and the US Food and Drugs Administration (FDA) the Multi-Item Gamma Poisson Shrinker (MGPS), both of which are more complex measures based on Bayesian statistics. These measures tend to produce less extreme values than PRRs when the number of cases is very small. However, when the sensitivity, specificity and predictive power of these measures were compared using Dutch data in 2002, no important differences were found provided at least three cases had been reported. In addition to PRRs, the UK regulatory authority now uses the empirical Bayes geometric mean (EBGM).

A number of points about these methods are worth emphasising. First, although the numbers are calculated in a similar way to relative risks, they do not represent a meaningful calculation of risk. While it is true that the greater the degree of disproportionality, the more reason there is to look further, the only real utility of the numbers is to decide whether there are more cases than might reasonably have been expected. Indicators of disproportionality are measures of association and even quite extreme results may not be causal. The next step is detailed clinical review of the relevant individual case reports and to assess any other relevant information which may be available. Many pharmacovigilance experts do not regard mathematical disproportionality alone as sufficient to raise a 'signal'. Thus, use of the terms 'statistical signal' and 'signal of disproportionate reporting' has emerged.

Aside from such semantic considerations, the underlying nature of the data and various potential biases inherent in spontaneous ADR reporting must not be forgotten. A specific problem arising from proportionate methods is that large effects may swamp and therefore mask smaller ones. For example, it is fairly obvious that PRRs calculated for all the other suspected reactions reported with rifabutin (the example given earlier) are going to be less than 1 but it is quite possible that some of these reactions would also be worth looking into further.

The data mining approach to signal detection has been questioned by some practitioners who believe that relying on clinical experience alone is preferable and that there are too many limitations to the disproportionality methods. It is generally agreed that detailed assessment of individual case reports (preferably by those with clinical experience) should be a key component of signal identification, but in databases where there are large numbers of ADRs, data mining may be seen as a useful first step to raise possible issues to examine further, or to add supporting evidence when assessing and investigating individual case reports. Hence, data mining should not be seen as a replacement for clinical assessment of reports, but rather an aid to it.

Evaluation and Investigation

Signal Prioritisation

Systematic use of data mining tools in a large spontaneous ADR database will identify large numbers of statistical signals. Evaluating all of them in detail would have major resource implications as many will turn out not to be real or to require no action. Possible signals have often been evaluated or dismissed on the basis of subjective judgements, but two more formal methods of prioritisation have been developed.

1) *Triage* (used by the WHO UMC) analogous to a process used in emergency medicine to decide on priorities. Essentially, it is a quick look at the most important features of a case series (e.g. seriousness, outcome) to decide on the urgency of further assessment relative to other cases.

2) *Impact analysis* (used by the UK MHRA) more quantitative and involves calculating two scores which are then used to decide an overall priority:
Evidence score:
- Based on the degree of disproportionality (e.g. value of PRR)
- Strength of evidence
- Biological plausibility.
Public health score:
- Based on number of reported cases per year
- Expected health consequences
- Reporting rate in relation to level of drug exposure.
The overall categories derived from these scores are as follows:
- High priority – prompt further evaluation is required
- Need to gather more information
- Low priority
- No action.

It is important to recognise that these scores are only a means of deciding whether further evaluation is currently warranted and that impact analysis can – and should be – repeated if more evidence emerges.

Principles of Signal Evaluation

The data giving rise to the signal – whether arising from a series of individual cases or a formal study – should be evaluated in detail first. It is also important to consider what other immediately available data might be relevant, to obtain them and to include them in the evaluation. For example, are there any other cases of the putative ADR (or similar clinical events) in randomised clinical trials, or are there any relevant pre-clinical findings? Are there any epidemiological data that might help, or is there anything of relevance in the published literature?

When evaluating a signal the key issues are:

- *Causality* – does the balance of evidence support cause and effect (see Chapter 2)?
- *Frequency* – if this is a real effect, how often is it occurring? Can we make any estimate of the likely level of absolute risk (see Chapter 2)?
- *Seriousness of the ADR* – are there any fatal cases, is the reaction potentially life-threatening, can it result in long-term disability?
- *Other clinical implications* – even if the ADR is not serious (as defined here and in Chapter 2), are there other important effects for patients and healthcare systems (e.g. need for extensive investigations or inability to work)?
- *Preventability* – are there any factors that, even at this stage, suggest a potential means to prevent the adverse reaction or serious outcomes arising from it?

In terms of frequency, the descriptors originally proposed by a CIOMS working group (see Chapter 6) are generally used, based on orders of magnitude and expressed as a simple proportion of patients affected (Table 4.2).

When evaluating signals from spontaneous reporting data, it is often difficult to obtain denominator or exposure data which are accurate enough to make a more precise estimate of expected ADR frequency than suggested earlier. We have already mentioned that sales data have limitations and provide only a rough estimate of usage.

Table 4.2 Descriptors originally proposed by a Council for International Organizations of Medical Sciences (CIOMS) working group.

CIOMS descriptor	Frequency
Very common	More than 1 in 10
Common	1 in 10 to 1 in 100
Uncommon	1 in 100 to 1 in 1000
Rare	1 in 1000 to 1 in 10 000
Very rare	Less than 1 in 10 000

The most accurate way to estimate frequency of ADRs in post-marketing use is from more formal pharmacoepidemiology studies, for example PEM studies (see Chapter 3) where cohorts of patients are established from prescription records.

The outcome of signal evaluation is often that there is a need for further investigation, but there can also be enough evidence and concern to take action without waiting for confirmatory studies. If several deaths or serious ADRs had been reported and causality assessment suggested a 'definite' or 'probable' relationship with a specific medicine (see Chapter 2), it would not be ethical to wait for more formal studies to be designed, conducted and analysed. Also, in some cases, it may not be feasible to conduct further studies because no suitable resource is available with data on enough patients.

Further Investigation

Primarily, signals are further investigated to provide more information about the key issues in signal evaluation – to try to gain better evidence on whether the drug really does cause the effect, how common it is, how serious it is and how it might be prevented. In respect of the latter, this is often a question of trying to identify who is at particular risk of the adverse effect (i.e. what are the risk factors?; this is discussed further in Chapter 7). Thus, as discussed in Chapter 3, pharmacoepidemiological studies are the main way in which signals are further investigated.

Another common avenue of investigation is through mechanistic studies (i.e. through the application of basic science in the laboratory, can we understand the biological mechanism of the ADR?) Knowing, for example, that an adverse effect mostly occurs in people who are poor metabolisers of specific hepatic cytochrome substrates could be important in developing preventive measures.

Taking Action

Potential Options

The ultimate purpose of pharmacovigilance is prevention and therefore the actions that are taken will generally be intended to help prevent occurrence of ADRs in the future. There are many factors that can impact on the potential for prevention of ADRs. Broadly, these can be classified into characteristics of the user or the drug:

1) *User characteristics:*
   - Demographics: age, sex, race
   - Genetic factors: polymorphisms (e.g. acetylator status)
   - Concomitant diseases (e.g. impaired hepatic or renal failure)
   - History of previous ADRs (e.g. allergy)
   - Compliance and use of other medicines.
2) *Drug characteristics:*
   - Route of administration
   - Formulation (e.g. sustained vs. immediate release, excipients)
   - Dosage regimen
   - Therapeutic index (a measure of the intrinsic safety of a drug in relation to dose)
   - Mechanisms of drug metabolism and route of excretion
   - Potential for drug interactions.

Based on these possibilities, a wide variety of potential actions can be considered and in various combinations. For taking regulatory action, it is useful to think of these in relation to the structure of the Summary of Product Characteristics (SPC), sections 4.1–4.9, and the potential amendments that might be made (Table 4.3). Thus, it can be seen that every section of the clinical advice in the SPC might potentially need to be modified in relation to a new drug safety issue.

Apart from amending the advice to users, there are two more drastic types of regulatory action that might be considered. The first is to take some steps, beyond mere recommendation, to ensure that a key part of advice is implemented in practice. The second is to remove the drug from the market. A good example of the former is the scheme that was set up to ensure that users of the antipsychotic drug clozapine have their white blood cell counts effectively monitored (see Chapter 7). In essence, further supply of the drug was linked to the availability of a blood test result (i.e. no blood, no drug). The reason for this was that it had been demonstrated that regular blood tests would generally pick up a falling white blood cell count before patients developed serious infections and also that on stopping the drug, the process was reversible. A further example of a scheme that takes active steps to ensure that measures necessary to minimise risks are taken by users are the pregnancy prevention programmes set up for users of isotretinoin (a known teratogen).

Table 4.3 Potential for actions to improve safety related to sections
of the Summary of Product Characteristics (SPC).

Section of SPC	Examples
Indications/uses	Limiting the indications to particular conditions with the greatest benefits by removal of indications: (a) for which the benefits are insufficient to justify use; (b) for which use is associated with a greater risk of the ADR
Dosing instructions	Reductions in dose (may be applied to specific groups, e.g. the elderly); limitations on duration or frequency of treatment (especially for ADRs related to cumulative dose); provision of information on safer administration
Contraindications	Addition of concomitant diseases and/or medications for which the risks of use are expected to outweigh the benefits
Warnings/ precautions	Addition of concomitant diseases and/or medications for which the risks of use need to be weighed carefully against the benefits; additional or modified recommendations for monitoring patients
Interactions	Addition of concomitant medications, alcohol or foods that may interact; advice on co-prescription and any monitoring required
Pregnancy/lactation	Addition of new information relating to effects on the fetus or neonate; revised advice about use in these circumstances based on accumulating experience or other new data
Effects on driving or using machinery	Practical advice on possible impairment of coordination or other effects due to ADRs such as sleepiness
Undesirable effects	Addition of newly recognised ADRs; improving information about the nature, frequency and severity of effects already listed
Overdosage	Adverse effects of overdosage; management, including the need for monitoring

In both these examples, the drugs appear to have particular benefits not shared by alternative treatments.

Over a period of many years, about 4% of drugs put on the market have had to be withdrawn for safety reasons – a fairly low proportion. This reflects reluctance to use this measure unless it is clear that, relative to alternative treatments, the risks outweigh the benefits despite maximum attempts to minimise the risks (and maximise the benefits).

Withdrawal from the market is particularly problematic for drugs that are used chronically by large numbers of patients. If the adverse effect tends to occur early in treatment, established users will have a relatively low risk of the ADR – the main need is to prevent new starters. Existing regulatory systems do not readily address this dilemma although in some instances it is possible for patients using a withdrawn medicine to continue it on a 'compassionate use' basis.

When considering such decisions in the face of uncertain data it may be necessary to take into account the impact of the *precautionary principle*. While, scientifically, it may seem unsatisfactory to act decisively on unconfirmed risks – the need being for more data – some decisions may have to be made in advance of definitive data, and the precautionary principle is well-established in many areas of regulation. In particular, patients should not be expected to take a possible additional risk when there is no evidence of possible advantage in doing so. On the other hand, removing a drug from the market may mean that it becomes almost impossible to study it further and that clear answers will never be forthcoming.

Making a Decision

The first step in making a decision about how to manage an important drug safety issue is to bring together all the relevant evidence into a single document. This is usually called a benefit–risk report and there is an internationally agreed structure which has been defined in a report published by the CIOMS IV working group (see Chapter 6). Both companies and regulatory authorities use the report format and both usually use experts, often in the form of a committee, to review the report and help formulate the decision. Lay representation on regulatory committees has become increasingly common as such decisions are not purely technical and scientific, they involve value judgements and consideration of the impact of such decisions on patients' lives. In most countries, regulatory decisions are overseen and sometimes directly made by politicians who are not necessarily bound by the scientific advice they receive.

The following is a suggested basic approach or framework for making decisions on drug safety (i.e. a structured list of the issues that should be taken into account):

1) What is the nature of problem?
2) What is the evidence of benefit?
3) What is the evidence for risk?

4) How strongly would we wish to avoid the risks and obtain the benefits in terms of the nature of the potential harms and expected positive effects?
5) What assumptions have we made and how valid are they?
6) What areas of uncertainty remain and what evidence is missing?
7) What are the options for action?
8) What are the expected consequences of each option?

Implementation

Unless the medicine is to be withdrawn from the market, most regulatory actions that could be taken will involve a change to the marketing authorisation and product information. Occasionally, the existing product information is considered satisfactory and the problem is merely that the recommendations within it are frequently not being followed. In these circumstances, 'reminder' communications may be issued, often directly by regulatory authorities and through regular bulletins by which the authorities communicate with health professionals. However, the extent to which these influence the behaviour of prescribers is unclear.

An important consideration is how quickly information needs to be made available to health professionals and patients. A new life-threatening ADR requires immediate communication, whereas the addition of a symptom that does not appear to be associated with serious consequences (e.g. nausea) to the undesirable effects section of the product information could be part of the next routine revision of the SPC. Most issues come between these two extremes and a judgement needs to be made about the speed of action and the most appropriate method of communication.

An issue that is particularly difficult relates to communication of signals to users of medicines. In the past, unconfirmed signals have rarely been communicated actively by regulatory bodies because of the uncertainty involved and because it is often difficult to make clear recommendations to users. However, in recent years expectations have changed and appearing to 'sit' on potentially worrying information which then leaks out can damage confidence in the system and lead to perceptions that the data are worse than is really the case. In an important example, in 2007 the WHO UMC published a signal of approximately 10-fold disproportionate ADR reporting identified from their spontaneous database related to statins and amyotrophic lateral sclerosis (a life-threatening neurological condition) despite much uncertainty about cause and effect. This was picked up and covered by the general media but, despite the very wide use of statins, it did not appear to create a major 'scare'. Subsequently, the signal was effectively disproved by further investigation. It is likely that information about signals will increasingly be actively communicated in the future, for example through social media.

Other Methods of Implementing Changes in Practice

Once a signal has been identified, it is primarily the responsibility of regulators to take action and implement changes in prescribing and use of medicines, using the methods described. However, this part of the pharmacovigilance process can also be supported and enhanced by other professional bodies, international organisations and also patient/consumer groups to achieve effective results. An example relates to the contraceptive device Implanon. In the early 2000s, more than 200 unintended pregnancies following insertion of Implanon devices were reported to the Australian national regulatory body, the Therapeutic Goods Adminstration (TGA). This signal was investigated by the TGA in collaboration with an academic researcher and published as a case series in 2006. It transpired that many of the devices had not been correctly inserted and changes were subsequently made to the Implanon product information. In addition to the work carried out by the TGA to resolve this issue, professional bodies in Australia assisted the sponsor company with providing additional training to inserters of Implanon. Following these actions, the numbers of unintended pregnancies with Implanon in Australia fell significantly.

Communication

Principles

Communication is a vital stage in the pharmacovigilance process, but one that is hard to get right, particularly if there is an urgent need to act. The example of oral contraceptives and 'pill scares' discussed in Chapter 1 led to much more attention to this aspect and discussion of the principles involved. Since the late 1990s, risk communication has developed as a sub-specialist area of pharmacovigilance (with an increasing number of publications in academic journals) and it is now recognised that a particular set of skills is required to achieve effective communication.

The main requirements for a successful drug safety communication are that it is accurate, balanced, open, understandable and targeted. These can be remembered by the mnemonic ABOUT (Table 4.4).

Practical Issues

The ABOUT criteria are considerations that can be used to formulate the process of developing a communication. A draft should be tested against these requirements by a review process which includes both individuals who are experts in the field and those who are generalists. Communications intended for patients should be written in plain language and reviewed by lay people. Information should be prepared in the appropriate languages of the target populations in the countries affected. In urgent situations it is vital to spend enough of the time that is available ensuring that these requirements are met.

Table 4.4 Key requirements for a successful drug safety communication (ABOUT).

Requirement	Comments
Accurate	Are the facts and numbers correct? Is all the information that the reader needs to know included?
Balanced	Have both risks and benefits been considered? Is the overall message right?
Open	Is the communication completely honest about the hazard without any attempt to hide or minimise it? Have any conflicts of interest been declared and explained?
Understandable	Should be as straightforward as possible using lay language without jargon – the reader is more likely to respond appropriately if the message is simple and clear
Targeted	This involves considering who is the intended audience and their specific information needs

It is particularly important in any communication about drug safety to ensure that essential information is clearly conveyed and not obscured by other less important information. The key facts and advice should be placed in a prominent early position (as many people will only read the first paragraph) with use of highlighting where needed. A clear lay-out with sub-headings, a large enough font, use of bolding/colour and inclusion of appropriate pictures or diagrams can make a huge difference to readability and effective communication. It is vital that the level of the risk is made very clear by expressing it in absolute rather than relative terms (see Chapter 2). The need for clear and simple language is vital – a good tip when drafting is to read the communication out loud and listen to how it sounds.

Table 4.5 represents a basic model for any drug safety communication, whether it is to be targeted at health professionals or at a lay audience (e.g. the general media).

Information sent to health professionals should be clearly labelled 'Important safety information' and, if appropriate, 'Urgent'. It is also useful to prepare answers to 'Frequently asked questions' as these are often placed on relevant websites.

Methods of Communication

Today there are many different ways in which drug safety messages can be conveyed to the target audience (which must be clearly defined), from hard copy letters through to electronic methods including social media and text messaging. It is important to consider which means will be most effective in the local environment and also which are the most appropriate. These aspects of risk communication are still evolving.

Table 4.5 Basic model for a drug safety communication.

Short heading which includes the drug and hazard

1) Nature of the problem: drug, hazard, precipitating factor(s)
2) Summary of the evidence for the hazard
3) What is being done: for example reviewing, investigating, new studies, changing labelling and so on
4) What are the implications for: (a) health professionals; (b) patients?
5) Overall balanced view of risks and benefits
6) Where to get further information/contact details

Measuring the Effectiveness of the Risk Minimisation Process

Measuring the success (or failure) of actions taken to minimise risk is an important step in the overall process, but one that is often overlooked or poorly done. Broadly, the possible methods of evaluating the effectiveness of actions taken are as follows:

- *Testing the effectiveness of the communications* – have they been received and understood (e.g. using market research techniques)?
- *Analysing the effect on prescribing* – the extent to which prescribing habits may have been modified and whether these changes consistent with revised recommendations in the product information (e.g. using longitudinal patient databases).
- *Monitoring spontaneously reported cases* – to see whether serious cases continue to be reported. The numbers of cases reported may be difficult to interpret because of publicity bias, but it can be useful to see, for example, whether any of the reported cases reflect contraindicated use.
- *Observation/formal study of prescribing and events* – has the action resulted in reduced morbidity/mortality from the ADR in practice? This will require use of a longitudinal patient database, performance of clinical audits or an epidemiological study. A formal pharmacoepidemiological study is perhaps the ideal but has been the least frequently undertaken of these activities.

Crisis Management

Every drug safety issue is different and an important step in dealing with one is to determine the level of urgency, using the principles discussed (broadly, the public health impact taking into account the absolute frequency of the hazard, number of users and seriousness). Major, newly identified hazards result in a need to re-evaluate the overall risk–benefit balance of a product. The highest level of urgency occurs when new evidence emerges suggesting that the risks of a medicine may outweigh the benefits, either for all users or in specific circumstances (e.g. a particular indication). Thus, a potential or defined need to withdraw a drug on safety grounds is inevitably a crisis situation for all those involved in its management. In these circumstances, any delay can result in damage to patients and reasonable haste is necessary.

Crisis management in drug safety is not fundamentally different from dealing with other types of crisis. A standard operating procedure for crisis management needs to be in place beforehand defining:

- What will be considered a crisis
- Composition of the crisis team and responsibilities
- Stakeholders and need for interactions with them.

The first task of the crisis team is to draw up a specific crisis management plan which will define the following:

- Key objectives
- Expected timelines (likely to be days to a few weeks at most)
- Resources required
- Responsibilities.

The key tasks for the drug safety crisis team are likely to be the following:

- Evaluation of the evidence
- Decision-making
- Practical arrangements for implementation
- Developing the external communication materials.

Progress towards the objectives needs to be reviewed daily and effective internal communication is vital. Because a regulatory authority or company (or other organisation) needs to deal with a crisis does not mean that routine work and other obligations can be ignored. Therefore, personnel who continue to deal with routine work should ideally be kept entirely separate from the crisis team.

Conclusions

This chapter has considered the process of pharmacovigilance from a signal of possible hazard through to remedial action, including effective risk communication. The outlined principles apply to pharmaceutical companies, regulatory authorities, researchers and other professionals involved in the practice of pharmacovigilance worldwide, including those who can support implementation of changes in clinical practice in order to achieve safer use of medicines. Good communication, both within organisations and with external stakeholders, is essential in achieving the best results from the process. Chapter 5 considers how companies and regulators should interact to ensure that the pharmacovigilance process is appropriately applied.

5

Regulatory Aspects of Pharmacovigilance

The need for medicines regulation and pharmacovigilance became widely recognised in the 1960s as a consequence of the thalidomide tragedy. The role of regulatory authorities worldwide is to protect public health by promoting the safe and effective use of medicines. In general terms, these activities are also in the interests of pharmaceutical companies, but industry has an additional, commercial driver – the needs to recoup investments in products and to satisfy shareholders. As health and financial drivers sometimes conflict, the authorities have compulsory powers to act on grounds of safety. However, these powers are only used when necessary and most of the time regulatory authorities seek and gain voluntary agreement from companies for the necessary measures.

Legally, both the authorities and manufacturers are responsible for the safety of medicinal products. In the European Union (EU), both parties are obliged to operate pharmacovigilance systems, to exchange data and, where necessary, to take appropriate action to protect patients. The responsibilities of the authorities generally cover all medicinal products – and there are many thousands of them. Therefore, in practice, they have to focus particularly on issues that are the most important for public health. As the early post-marketing phase is invariably a period of considerable uncertainty about safety and the time when important new hazards are most likely to be identified, most regulatory pharmacovigilance activity is concentrated on newer drugs.

In this chapter, 'regulation' is considered from both sides of the fence: that is, from the perspective of both the regulator and industry. The regulatory obligations of pharmaceutical companies are

An Introduction to Pharmacovigilance, Second Edition. Patrick Waller and Mira Harrison-Woolrych.

extensively laid out in legislation and guidelines, but it is important to appreciate that merely meeting these obligations does not ensure the safety of medicinal products. Rather, they should be seen as an essential baseline from which an acceptable safety standard can potentially be achieved. Since the beginning of the twenty-first century it has been formally recognised that the whole process was previously too passive, that more and better post-authorisation safety studies are needed, and that proper planning is required if adequate safety knowledge is to be gained. This has led to the introduction of risk management planning to underpin the whole process.

Legislation and Guidelines

Despite ongoing attempts at international harmonisation (see Chapter 6), legislative requirements for the regulation of medicines continue to differ around the world. Most countries have a medicines regulatory body, which usually operates from within the relevant government department. Pharmaceutical companies are obliged to submit applications to it in territories in which they wish to market their products. In this section, we focus on the EU where, as in many countries around the world, medicines legislation is supported by guidance to give practical advice on how to comply with the law. Following guidelines is generally a good practice, but it may not always be possible or appropriate. Guidelines are much more easily amended than legislation and tend to increase in size as issues of interpretation are addressed.

Key Elements of European Legislation

EU medicines legislation has two broad aims: protection of public health and the creation of a single market for pharmaceuticals. EU legislation is initially proposed by the European Commission, goes through extensive consultative and political processes and emerges via the European Parliament to be put into force by the Commission. In principle, if there is an apparent conflict with any national legislation, EU law takes precedence. However, this does not necessarily mean that national authorities cannot enforce additional requirements in their own territory. A centralised system of authorisation (i.e. one licence valid throughout the EU) was introduced in 1995 and in recent years its use has been obligatory for all new drugs. Many older products have national authorisations in some individual or all Member States. For such medicines, product information may still differ, but when important safety issues arise procedures are available to ensure that harmonised action is taken across the EU.

The legislation defining the centralised system of authorisation is in the form of Regulations, which are directly effective in all Member States. Other relevant EU legislation is contained in Directives, which oblige Member States to implement national laws having specified effects. Until 2010, EU pharmacovigilance legislation occupied short sections within each of the broad legislative documents covering medicines regulation in general:

- Regulation 2309/93, articles 19–26
- Directive 2001/83, Title IX, articles 101–108.

These articles briefly defined the need for both Member States and pharmaceutical companies to operate pharmacovigilance systems and were largely focused on adverse reaction reporting systems. They were supported by quite extensive guidance which had been developed over many years and was known as Volume 9A.

In 2010, after extensive consultation and development, two major pieces of pharmacovigilance legislation were enacted and came into force in mid-2012:

- Regulation 2010/1235, and
- Directive 2010/84

which amend the previous Regulation and Directive to introduce substantial new requirements, and greatly increase the volume of pharmacovigilance legislation. There is also an implementing Regulation 520/2012 which covers various practical aspects of the regulatory pharmacovigilance process, for example the contents of key documents such as the pharmacovigilance system master file, risk management plan and periodic safety update report.

The 'recitals' at beginning of the main new legislation explain the reasoning behind it and define three broad objectives:

1) Strengthen post-authorisation regulation of medicines
2) Improve efficiency, both within the pharmaceutical industry and through reduced duplication of effort between the Member States
3) Increase transparency.

To underpin these developments, a Pharmacovigilance Risk Assessment Committee (PRAC) was formed consisting of representatives of Member States, healthcare professionals, patient organisations and independent experts. It meets monthly at the European Medicines Agency (EMA). The pharmacovigilance legislation that came into effect in 2012 also mandated the development of good pharmacovigilance practice (GVP) to replace existing guidance.

When required, regulatory action is taken through the European or national marketing authorisations. The options available are suspension, revocation or variation. These powers are specified in article 116 of Directive 2001/83 (which is not part of the section on pharmacovigilance) and an unfavourable risk–benefit balance (section 117 (c)) provides the most usual basis for compulsory withdrawal from the market. Suspension is temporary and usually put in place as a matter of urgency. Revocation leads to permanent removal of the product and this decision is taken over a longer time scale. In either case, the marketing authorisation (MA) holder is usually given the opportunity to make representations to the authorities. As discussed in Chapter 4, variation of the authorisation is the most common mechanism for dealing with pharmacovigilance issues and, if urgent, there is a mechanism for making safety restrictions within 24 hours. Both the authorities and companies can initiate such restrictions.

Aside from the above legislation, the Regulation covering clinical trials (Regulation 2014/536) is relevant to pharmacovigilance for investigational drugs (i.e. those that are not yet authorised) and Annex 3 specifies the safety reporting requirements.

The most important principles specified in the EU legislation that came into effect in 2012 can be summarised as follows:

- Pharmacovigilance is based largely on existing national systems.
- Member States are responsible for conducting pharmacovigilance in their own territories.
- The EMA is responsible for coordination, and maintenance of (a) the central pharmacovigilance database (EudraVigilance) and (b) a web portal, the purpose of which is to promote transparency in pharmacovigilance by disseminating defined information about medicines authorised in the EU.
- The key advisory forum is the PRAC on whose recommendations the handling of pharmacovigilance issues is based.
- MA holders have defined responsibilities.

Guidelines

Over the past few years, EU guidance has been extensively changed by the genesis of GVP. As with legislation, there are consultation processes involved in the development of guidelines. At the time of writing, 12 modules of GVP have been developed and published on the EMA's website (Box 5.1). The titles of these modules are shown in Table 5.1. As well as the general procedural considerations addressed by these guidance documents, a GVP series addressing product or population-specific considerations is being developed with chapters relating to: (i) vaccines, (ii) biologicals, (iii) pregnancy and breast feeding, (iv) children and (v) the elderly, either published or in preparation.

There is additional pharmacovigilance guidance on the EMA website which is not part of GVP. For example, these cover requirements specific to the centralised system and provide questions and answers in relation to company pharmacovigilance systems. Also relevant to pharmacovigilance are guidelines on the Summary of Product Characteristics (SPC) and Package Leaflet (in Volume 2 of the Rules Governing Medicinal Products), and, for investigational drugs, clinical trial guidelines (Volume 10 of the Rules Governing Medicinal Products, Chapter II). These are part of Eudralex and can be found in the public health section of the European Commission's website (Box 5.1).

Box 5.1 Key website references.

EudraVigilance: http://www.ema.europa.eu/ema/index.jsp?curl=pages/regulation/general/general_content_000679.jsp&mid=WC0b01ac05800250b5

European Commission's legislation pages (Eudralex): http://ec.europa.eu/health/documents/eudralex/index_en.htm

European Medicines Agency's Good Pharmacovigilance Practice pages: http://www.ema.europa.eu/ema/index.jsp?curl=pages/regulation/document_listing/document_listing_000345.jsp&mid=WC0b01ac058058f32c

European Network of Centres for Pharmacoepidemiology and Pharmacovigilance: www.encepp.eu

Table 5.1 Good pharmacovigilance practice (GVP) Modules.

No.	Title
I	Pharmacovigilance systems and their quality systems
II	Pharmacovigilance system master file
III	Pharmacovigilance inspections
IV	Pharmacovigilance audits
V	Risk management systems
VI	Management and reporting of adverse reactions to medicinal products
VII	Periodic safety update report
VIII	Post-authorisation safety studies
IX	Signal management
X	Additional monitoring
XV	Safety communication
XVI	Risk minimisation measures – selection of tools and effectiveness indicators

Addenda

Module VI	Addendum I	Duplicate management of adverse reaction reports
Module VIII	Addendum I	Member States' requirements for transmission of information on non-interventional post-authorisation safety studies
Module XVI	Addendum I	Educational materials

Note: The following GVP Modules were originally planned but are no longer considered necessary given that other guidance has since been made available: Module XI on public participation; Module XII on safety-related action; Module XIII on incident management and exchange of information exchange within the EU regulatory network; and Module XIV on international collaboration.

Source: Produced from material published on the European Medicines Agency's website (© EMA [1995–2016]).

Regulatory Pharmacovigilance Systems

Broadly, there are two functions to pharmacovigilance from the perspective of a regulator: (i) the protection of public health by measures to promote safe and effective use of medicines and prevent serious adverse drug reactions (ADRs), and (ii) regulation of the industry.

Medicines regulatory authorities do not regulate health professionals, who are potentially able to prescribe medicines outside the terms of the authorisation (and unlicensed medicines) on their own responsibility.

In terms of protecting public health, regulators are active at every stage of the pharmacovigilance process described in Chapter 4: in the regulatory environment this means from the time a new medicine starts being studied in humans, through to post-marketing surveillance, which may continue for many years. In particular, regulators are concerned to ensure that signals are identified as rapidly as possible and are appropriately managed. They also aim to ensure that any actions taken are appropriate, communicated effectively and that their impact is measured.

In terms of regulating industry, the principal issue is one of compliance with the legal requirements. Formal monitoring of industry compliance with pharmacovigilance obligations through inspections is a fairly recent development. These inspections may be undertaken routinely, or at any time if the authorities have a reason to believe there may be non-compliance. There is a three-level approach to dealing with non-compliance. Relatively minor transgressions can be dealt with by educative measures or, in more serious cases, warnings are issued. In very serious or persistent cases, prosecution can be undertaken against the marketing authorisation holder. Offences are determined nationally but include substantial fines and even imprisonment, with both the company and the qualified person (see Company Pharmacovigilance Systems) being held responsible.

It should also be noted that regulators have obligations towards industry, in particular the timely availability to the MA holder of spontaneous ADR reports which they receive from health professionals. This is facilitated through the EudraVigilance database (Box 5.1). They are also obliged to audit their pharmacovigilance systems.

In order to provide the particular focus on new drugs alluded to, in 2013, EU regulators introduced an additional monitoring scheme which was mandated in the legislation. This is primarily for new drugs and usually lasts for 5 years after first authorisation. In order to promote ADR reporting for these products, they are identified by a black triangle symbol in the product information. This is essentially a modification of a scheme that has been in use in the UK since the 1980s.

The EMA publishes on its website lists of products under additional monitoring and, as well as new drugs, the lists include established ones with new safety concerns which are under investigation (e.g. domperidone, see example given later).

Obligations of Pharmaceutical Companies

Broadly, the pharmacovigilance obligations of companies can be summarised as follows:

- To operate a pharmacovigilance system with documented procedures (known as the pharmacovigilance system master file) and to regularly audit it
- To nominate a qualified person for pharmacovigilance
- ADR reporting
- Periodic safety update reporting
- To inform regulatory authorities of any information that may change the risk–benefit balance of a specific product
- To respond to requests for information from regulatory authorities
- To maintain a system to manage and minimise risk(s) with their medicines
- To keep the product information (including Patient Information Leaflets, PILs) up-to-date
- To comply with regulations for marketing and advertising pharmaceutical products.

Company Pharmacovigilance Systems

The qualified person for pharmacovigilance (QPPV) takes personal responsibility for organisation and management of the pharmacovigilance system within the company. They need to be always available and therefore most large companies also nominate a deputy. It is essential that documented quality procedures are put in place in the form of a pharmacovigilance system master file. Effective pharmacovigilance requires a properly functioning database containing accurate up-to-date data. All personnel within the department must be appropriately trained. General system compliance with these principles is now monitored by regulatory authorities through inspections.

ADR Reporting

We have described the principles of spontaneous ADR reporting in Chapter 3 and how the data are used in the pharmacovigilance process in Chapter 4. Next, we consider the principal activities undertaken by company pharmacovigilance departments: ADR reporting, periodic safety update reporting, post-authorisation safety studies and risk management planning. It should be self-evident that the purpose of company ADR reporting obligations is to ensure that regulators have prompt access to reports which are submitted directly to companies. This led to the concept of the 'expedited' report – in essence this is a report of a serious (as defined in Chapter 1) suspected ADR and the obligation is to submit it to the authorities within 15 calendar days of receipt. Non-serious reports should be submitted within 90 days. In the EU, the use of the Medical Dictionary for Regulatory Affairs (MedDRA) for coding is mandatory and reporting electronically via EudraVigilance is expected to become mandatory for MA holders in 2017.

EudraVigilance is the EU regulatory network's system for managing information on suspected ADRs reported with authorised medicines, managed by the EMA. It supports safety monitoring by facilitating the electronic exchange of suspected ADR reports among the EMA, national competent authorities, MA holders and sponsors of clinical trials.

The principal use of EudraVigilance is in the early detection and evaluation of possible safety signals for human medicines. It includes an automated message processing mechanism and a large pharmacovigilance database with query, tracking and tracing capabilities. The EMA publishes data from EudraVigilance as the European database of suspected ADR reports. A public website allows users to view the numbers of serious individual case reports submitted to EudraVigilance for centrally authorised medicines. On their website, the EMA also publishes reports for common drug substances contained in nationally authorised medicines.

There are two further important principles for pharmaceutical companies. The first is that *serious* (see Glossary) and fatal reports should be followed-up and the information obtained also reported within 15 days. Companies should also follow-up incomplete ADR reports and any that represent an event of special interest for the product concerned (e.g. reports of pregnancy for a medicine that is used in women of reproductive age). Secondly, companies should be proactive in searching the medical literature, media (including social media) and the internet to identify potential case reports of ADRs that are not well recognised to occur with their drugs. Assuming they are valid and have been assessed by the company as serious, these should also be submitted within 15 days. A valid individual case safety report meets four criteria:

1) At least one identifiable reporter
2) One single identifiable patient
3) At least one suspected adverse reaction and
4) At least one suspected medicinal product.

Prior to authorisation, in relation to products being investigated in clinical trials, ADR reporting requirements are different. The key principles here are that *serious and unexpected* (meaning not listed in the Investigator's Brochure for that specific trial) suspected ADRs (SUSARs) should be expedited, and that such reports should be unblinded for this purpose. Steps should be taken to ensure that personnel directly involved in the trial remain blinded. Companies are required to submit SUSARs both to regulatory authorities and to the ethics committee(s) that approved the trial. They must also ensure that all investigators are kept informed about SUSARs so as to meet the key objective of protecting the safety of trial participants.

The practice of ADR reporting by companies has many complexities which are best learned 'on the job' and by applying the available regulatory guidelines. These principles give an overview of current practice and it is the responsibility of industry to keep up-to-date with changing guidance and discuss cases of doubt with the relevant regulatory authority.

Periodic Safety Update Reporting

The concept of, and format for, periodic safety update reporting was developed in the early 1990s by the Council for International Organizations of Medical Sciences (CIOMS) working group (see Chapter 6) and rapidly implemented into legislation in many parts of the world. The objective of producing Periodic Safety Update Reports (PSURs) is to facilitate regular, systematic review of the *global* safety data available to the manufacturer of marketed products. Over time, the scope of the PSUR has tended to broaden and the overall goal of such review is to identify any change in the *benefit–risk* profile of the product that might require further investigation or action. Following the adoption of International Council on Harmonisation of Technical Requirements for Pharmaceuticals for Human Use (ICH) guideline E2C (see Chapter 6), PSURs are now also known as Periodic Benefit–Risk Evaluation Reports (PBRERs), reflecting this broadened scope from safety to benefit–risk.

Production of PSURs starts when a drug is first approved for marketing anywhere in the world (international birth date, IBD) and, initially, reports are produced on a 6-monthly basis. The period covered becomes longer once the drug is established in the market but precise requirements have varied over time and between countries. In the EU, the new legislation seeks to make the requirements proportionate to the risks. For example, it no longer routinely requires PSURs for generic products containing drugs the safety of which is well established.

The main body of data in each PSUR covers a defined period of time, starting either at the IBD or when data for the previous report were 'locked' (i.e. the point at which further information received cannot be included in the report). The contents and structure of a PSUR is summarised in Table 5.2. The 'reference' or 'core' safety information is also included as an appendix. This is a minimum standard of information which is considered essential for safe use and will be included in all product information worldwide.

Key sections of the PSUR are those that evaluate signals, the integrated risk–benefit evaluation and the overall conclusions and actions proposed. These sections are where any important newly identified or ongoing safety issues are assessed and proposals made to address them.

PSURs are routinely reviewed by regulatory authorities around the world. In the EU, they are submitted in electronic format and the EMA undertakes a single assessment which is reviewed by the PRAC who make recommendations for any action to be taken through the MA. Meeting all the global requirements is complex and resource intensive, despite a fair degree of harmonisation. A format for safety update reporting in relation to investigational drugs in development (Development Safety Update Report, DSUR) has also been proposed by CIOMS (see Chapter 6), and adopted internationally. In the EU, guidance suggests that DSURs should be submitted annually to regulatory authorities.

Table 5.2 Structure of the Periodic Safety Update Report (PSUR).

Executive Summary	
1	Introduction
2	Worldwide marketing authorisation status
3	Actions taken in the reporting interval for safety reasons
4	Changes to reference safety information
5	Estimated exposure and use patterns
6	Data in summary tabulations
7	Summaries of significant findings from clinical trials during the reporting interval
8	Findings from non-interventional studies
9	Information from other clinical trials and sources
10	Non-clinical data
11	Literature
12	Other periodic reports
13	Lack of efficacy in controlled clinical trials
14	Late-breaking information
15	Overview of signals: new, ongoing or closed
16	Signal and risk evaluation
17	Benefit evaluation
18	Integrated benefit–risk analysis for authorised indications
19	Conclusions and actions
20	Appendices

Source: produced from material published on the European Medicines Agency's website (© EMA [1995–2016]).

Post-authorisation Safety Studies

Companies started to conduct these studies in the 1980s, but in the early days they were often seen as covert marketing exercises intended to promote use of a new medicine. Of course, it is impossible to study safety in ordinary practice if a drug is little used, but nevertheless it is important that post-marketing studies have clear safety objectives and do not interfere with prescribing practice. The emergence of databases such as the Clinical Practice Research Datalink in the

UK has lessened the need for studies that start by recruiting prescribing doctors and build up a cohort of users (see Chapter 3). From a scientific point of view, single cohort studies based on use of a particular drug have some limitations. They can measure the frequency of a particular event, but they may not provide any indication of the expected or background frequency, leading to judgements about causality being made from the individual cases. This problem is best addressed by including a comparison cohort of patients using an alternative treatment.

A frequent limitation of post-authorisation safety studies (PASS) is the sample size. Historically, 10 000 patients has often been a fairly arbitrary target for a drug that is likely to be widely used – this is based on the notion that it is about one order of magnitude more than the average number of patients studied in clinical trials. In terms of studying ADRs, which are rare or very rare, this will mean that there are only likely to be a few or possibly no cases observed in the study. In general, such studies will measure events rather than suspected ADRs, but any serious events that are suspected by investigators to be drug-related should be submitted to regulatory authorities as an expedited report.

Companies undertaking PASS will need to submit a draft protocol for review and endorsement by PRAC. They will also need to plan to provide data from the study to the regulatory authorities. The need for undertaking such studies will usually be specified in the risk management plan for the product (see Risk Management Planning). As well as studying ADRs, PASS can provide valuable information about drug utilisation. Who is using a medicine – and how – is an extremely important component of safety.

In recent years, the EMA has overseen the development of the European Network of Centres for Pharmacoepidemiology and Pharmacovigilance (ENCePP). Members of this network are public institutions and contract and research organisations involved in research in pharmacoepidemiology and pharmacovigilance. Research interests are not restricted to the safety of medicines, but include the benefits and risks of medicines, disease epidemiology and drug utilisation. ENCePP states that its aims are to strengthen the monitoring of the benefit–risk balance of medicinal products in Europe by:

- Facilitating the conduct of high quality, multi-centre, independent post-authorisation studies with a focus on observational research.

- Bringing together expertise and resources in pharmacoepidemiology and pharmacovigilance across Europe and providing a platform for collaborations.
- Developing and maintaining methodological standards and governance principles for research in pharmacovigilance and pharmacoepidemiology.

ENCePP has produced publicly accessible resources which include a database of available European research resources, a register of post-authorisation studies, a code of conduct which aims to promote transparency and scientific independence and guidance on methodological standards in pharmacoepidemiology.

An example of an important study undertaken through ENCePP is one that was undertaken to assess the rare risk of sudden cardiac death in association with domperidone, a drug widely used for gastro-intestinal symptoms such as nausea and vomiting. This *case–control study* (see Glossary) found an approximately twofold increased relative risk of sudden cardiac death which appeared to be dose-related. In 2014, taken in conjunction with other relevant data, the results of this study led PRAC to recommend restrictions on its use, strengthened warnings (particularly in relation to use of interacting drugs) and revocation of the MA for high dose products. In the UK, action was also taken to make the drug a prescription-only medicine.

Risk Management Planning

In the past, the pharmacovigilance process often lacked a clear starting point and an active plan to gain further safety knowledge and minimise risks. In recent years, considerable efforts have been made by regulatory authorities and companies to improve existing systems of risk management. It is now recognised that there is a need to focus more on safety, rather than harm, and to actively plan to demonstrate the safety of newly authorised products. An important development introduced into European regulatory processes in 2005 is risk management planning. In the EU, submission of a risk management plan (RMP) is now required with all new applications for MAs (not only all new active substances, but also generic products for example) and for changes to existing authorisations that are likely to significantly extend usage of the product. Plans may also be requested by the authorities at a later stage if an important new safety issue emerges.

The basic structure of an EU RMP, as defined the relevant GVP module, is shown in Table 5.3. The RMP should contain three key sections:

1) Safety specification
2) Pharmacovigilance plan
3) Risk minimisation plan.

The purpose of the safety specification is explicitly to consider the level of safety that has been demonstrated so far. It should identify what is and what *is not* yet known about safety and the latter (i.e. what is not known) should be a major driver of the pharmacovigilance plan. The purpose of that plan is essentially to attempt to find out what is not yet known, largely because of the limitations of clinical trials.

Table 5.3 Structure of an EU risk management plan.

Part I	Product(s) overview
Part II	Safety specification
	Epidemiology of the indication(s) and target population(s)
	Non-clinical part of the safety specification
	Clinical trial exposure
	Populations not studied in clinical trials
	Post-authorisation experience
	Additional EU requirements for the safety specification
	Identified and potential risks
	Summary of the safety concerns
Part III	Pharmacovigilance plan
Part IV	Plans for post-authorisation efficacy studies
Part V	Risk minimisation measures (including evaluation of the effectiveness of risk minimisation measures)
Part VI	Summary of the risk management plan
Part VII	Annexes

Source: produced from material published on the European Medicines Agency's website (© EMA [1995–2016]).

RMPs should be particularly focused on known or potential risks that cannot simply be managed through routine measures described in the product information.

Until recently, post-marketing safety activities in pharmaceutical companies mainly concerned satisfying the regulatory requirements outlined earlier in this chapter (i.e. spontaneous reporting and periodic safety update reports). While these are important, they do not in themselves ensure that medicines are safe and often they do little to demonstrate safety. They may also encourage a tendency towards focusing on bureaucratic requirements rather than public health. As it is impossible to know that a medicine is acceptably safe until it has been used in ordinary practice, it is reasonable to argue that demonstrating safety should be a key goal in the post-marketing period and therefore logical that it is necessary to plan how to achieve it.

Safety Specification

In the rest of the chapter we consider the key principles on which the key parts of the RMP are based. Any new medicine that has been authorised can be considered to have a level of safety which, in relation to its potential benefits and the disease being treated, is *provisionally* acceptable. The safety specification section of the RMP should document the basis of this judgement by considering the five broad areas set out next. The best starting point conceptually is to consider the disease that is to be treated or prevented and the characteristics of the target population.

Epidemiology of the Indication(s)

This should include the descriptive epidemiology of the disease indication(s): incidence, prevalence and demographic considerations, prognosis, likely co-morbidity and co-prescribing, plus medical events associated with the indication that could be mistaken for ADRs. Such information will be helpful for setting spontaneous ADR reports in context.

Extent of Current Clinical Safety Experience

This can be summarised in the form of graphs or tabulations, with calculations of the statistical power to detect ADRs according to duration of treatment and potential latency (i.e. time to onset), based on the following information:

- Overall numbers of patients studied for various durations of treatment and lengths of follow-up in all pre-marketing trials.
- Numbers of patients in different sub-groups, for example, split by age, gender, dose and other characteristics relevant to the disease being treated (presented by duration of treatment and length of follow-up). Both overall numbers (and sub-groups where feasible) are best shown graphically using plots of exposure over time (Figure 5.1).

Confirmed Adverse Reactions

The main focus here should be on ADRs identified in clinical trials described and quantified by system organ class. Analyses should be based on statistically significant differences seen between treated and control groups. This may be best presented as absolute excess risks with 95% confidence intervals.

Signals of Potential Adverse Reactions

These might include the following:

- Serious events that are not statistically significantly different between groups in clinical trials, but that constitute potential signals requiring further evaluation, based on a relative risk of at least 2 or

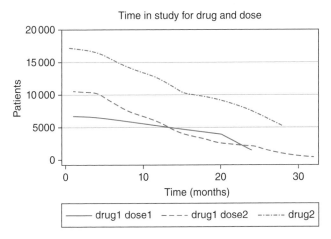

Figure 5.1 Drug exposure versus time, demonstrating the usual situation that, while quite large numbers of patients are exposed in pre-marketing trials for a few months, very few have been observed for more than 2 years.

at least one case that was thought to be related to the medicine (either by the investigator or the company following a formal causality assessment).

- Unconfirmed signals of potential toxicity (e.g. potential teratogenicity) found in pre-clinical data.

Areas of Safety Knowledge that are Incomplete
The main areas that are relevant here are:

- Special populations not studied in clinical trials (unless these are to be absolute contraindications to use of the drug), where experience is limited (e.g. children, pregnant women) or for which the safety profile might be expected to be different.
- Rare ADRs not yet observed with the drug, but which are recognised to occur with other drugs in the class, or which are possible based on knowledge of the molecular structure.
- Consideration of the potential for safety concerns based on off-label use, medication errors and intentional overdose.

Pharmacovigilance Plan

The marketing of a medicine represents both an opportunity and a need to demonstrate an acceptable level of safety. The pharmacovigilance plan should indicate how this will be achieved in practice, covering both routine pharmacovigilance activities (i.e. those required in legislation for all medicines) and any additional activities that are specific to the product (e.g. PASS). The plan might contain the following types of information:

- Expected levels of use of the product over time (worldwide)
- Strategies to address existing and potential safety signals
- Strategies to monitor recognised serious ADRs to ensure that their incidence is not greater than expected
- Strategies to address areas where safety knowledge is incomplete, for example in special populations
- Proposed milestones at which a greater level of safety experience is expected to have been demonstrated.

Most safety milestones (e.g. PSURs) are based on arbitrary measures of time. When they are reached, safety knowledge may or may not have been extended, in part depending on the level of usage of the product. A conceptually more logical way of defining milestones would be to base them on levels of exposure to the product. They can be derived using the expected level of use, taking into account power calculations indicating the known level of safety at authorisation. Milestones would then be reached when a specified number of patients had been studied (possibly for a specified length of time) or when particular safety studies are complete.

Risk Minimisation Plans

RMPs are particularly important when product information alone (i.e. SPC and PIL) is considered to provide insufficient safeguards against known or serious potential hazards. The additional risk minimisation measures that may be contained within them vary from providing general education (e.g. 'Dear Health Professional' communications) through specific training of users in safe administration, to restrictions on use-linked documentation of safe practice (e.g. ensuring that users of clozapine actually have acceptable white cell counts before a further prescription can be dispensed). There may also be additional risk minimisation measures for specific medicines or populations, for example pregnancy prevention programmes for medicines known to be teratogenic and likely to be used by women of childbearing potential (e.g. isotretinoin).

Whatever level of activity is envisioned, good communication is essential and it is important to consider and test the feasibility of the proposed measures. The most common form of activity is promotion of safe use and it is important that this is not confused with mere promotion of use. Regulators generally expect there to be clear daylight between the two activities and are unlikely to accept company representatives as the only vehicle for delivery of risk minimisation measures.

The final step in the process of pharmacovigilance is to assess the extent to which risk minimisation has been successful and if, necessary, to refine or change the measures. This is something that in the past has generally not been performed well, but is now part of the legislation and is receiving much more attention from the authorities.

Potential methods for measuring the success of risk minimisation (see Chapter 4 for further details) include:

- Testing the effectiveness of the communications
- Analysing the effects on prescribing

- Monitoring spontaneously reported cases
- Formal studies of measurable outcomes (e.g. analysing rates of ADRs in defined patient cohorts before and after risk minimization measures).

Simply monitoring spontaneous ADR reports is normally insufficient for the purpose of studying the effects of risk minimisation, but much can be learned from studies of drug utilisation and in particular from studying the characteristics of users and how a medicine is used. It is relatively easy, for example, to use a prescription database to examine concomitant use of interacting drugs, which might perhaps be contraindicated. Ideally, studies should measure hard and quantifiable outcomes, so that we can learn whether ADRs are being prevented by the measures put in place.

Conclusions

In this chapter, we have outlined the principles underpinning regulatory pharmacovigilance, focusing on the EU. Legally, both the regulatory authorities and manufacturers are responsible for the safety of medicinal products. Both are obliged to operate pharmacovigilance systems and, where necessary, to take appropriate action to protect patients. Key elements of the process are ADR reporting, periodic safety update reporting, PASS and risk management planning. Much of what we have described in this chapter relating to the EU has been developed through wider international cooperation. How and why this has happened, and the roles of the relevant international bodies is described in the next chapter.

6

International Collaboration

Pharmaceuticals are used by patients worldwide so global pharma-covigilance activities are needed to monitor the safety of medicines in all countries where they are marketed. There are many reasons for apparent international variations in the safety of medicines. The population in which a drug is used might be different in terms of ethnicity, demographic factors or the indication(s) for use. The need for a specific medicine and the way in which it might be used may differ (e.g. in terms of dose or monitoring), as might perceptions of risks and benefits in relation to alternative treatments. Despite the legitimacy of all such possible reasons, historical variations in safety recommendations and practice have undoubtedly exceeded what can be explained by them. There are many examples of drugs withdrawn or restricted in one part of the world remaining available in another for no rational reason. Such irrational international variations reflect uncertainty in the relevant data or differing views of experts who advise regulatory authorities on safety. In order to achieve patient safety across the globe – and consistency in practice – it has long been recognised that international harmonisation and cooperation are very important aspects of pharmacovigilance.

International collaboration in pharmacovigilance has advanced greatly in recent years. In medicines regulation, authorities around the world increasingly communicate about global regulatory issues and the pharmaceutical industry has been proactive in requesting international harmonisation for many processes, including adverse drug reaction (ADR) reporting. Non-governmental international organisations such as the World Health Organization (WHO), the Council for International Organizations of Medical Sciences (CIOMS)

An Introduction to Pharmacovigilance, Second Edition. Patrick Waller and Mira Harrison-Woolrych.
© 2017 John Wiley & Sons Ltd. Published 2017 by John Wiley & Sons Ltd.

and the International Council on Harmonisation (ICH) have continued to develop important pharmacovigilance services and guidelines on practice. Professional bodies – such as the International Society of Pharmacovigilance (ISoP) and the International Society for Pharmacoepidemiology (ISPE) – have become more global. In this chapter we give an overview of the activities and roles of the key international pharmacovigilance organisations and describe how they have developed and collaborated.

International Regulatory Collaboration

In Chapter 5 we described medicines regulation in the EU, with respect to pharmacovigilance. By developing centralised and harmonised processes, the European Medicines Agency (EMA) has addressed many differences in pharmacovigilance practice which previously existed between different member states – for example, products that had been withdrawn for safety reasons in one country, but not in another. The EMA has also developed centralised databases for ADR reporting, European guidelines on pharmacovigilance practice and expert advisory committees with representatives from all Member States (see Chapter 5). In these ways, the EMA has put international collaboration into active regulatory practice.

Outside Europe, most developed nations – and an increasing number of emerging and low and middle income countries – have their own medicines regulatory body. Countries with authorities covering the highest population size in the WHO Programme for International Drug Monitoring (WHO-PIDM) include those in Africa (e.g. Nigeria), the Middle East (e.g. Egypt), Asia (e.g. India, China and Japan), Central America (e.g. Mexico), South America (e.g. Brazil) and the Russian Federation. In most countries, pharmacovigilance activities are conducted by the national regulatory authority, which usually sits within the government's health department. However, there are notable exceptions, including in Japan, Korea, the Netherlands and New Zealand, where the pharmacovigilance centre lies outside the government regulatory body, collecting and providing data for the national authority.

The US Food and Drug Administration (FDA) is the oldest regulatory authority in the world. The FDA was established in 1906 and their remit has always included monitoring the safety of medicines and food products. This remains a key difference between the FDA and some other national regulatory authorities, including the UK

Medicines and Healthcare products Regulatory Agency (MHRA), which does not cover food (this is monitored by another UK government agency). However, many other national regulatory authorities (including several Asian authorities; for example, China FDA, Thai FDA, Philippines FDA) regulate food products in addition to drugs. The US FDA covers vaccines, blood products, medical devices, tobacco products, cosmetics and veterinary products, and so has a very wide scope.

By 2010, the US FDA employed nearly 15 000 people and in 2012 its annual budget was over $4 billion. The size and resources of the US FDA enabled it to lead the way in medicines regulation worldwide for many years, especially licensing of new medicines. Today, most other countries have their own regulatory authority but many countries still follow guidance developed in Europe (see Chapter 5) or the USA. Regarding pharmacovigilance, the FDA's primary tool is its spontaneous reporting programme, MedWatch, which was established in 1993. In more recent years, the FDA's requirements for post-marketing risk management have been increasing, as in Europe (see Chapter 5). In 2007, US legislation was amended, mainly as a consequence of concerns about rofecoxib (see Chapter 1) and the following year the FDA launched the Sentinel Initiative, a proactive electronic system for post-marketing surveillance.

In 2014, the UK MHRA and US FDA led discussions to establish a global regulatory authority which resulted in the formation of the International Coalition of Medicines Regulatory Authorities (ICMRA). The purpose of this voluntary organisation is to allow the heads of national regulatory authorities around the world to develop shared strategic leadership in order to address current and emerging global regulatory challenges, including safety issues. An example of this is that the ICMRA collaborated with the WHO in 2015 to help deal with the Ebola virus outbreak which affected many countries. The ICMRA has set up several working groups to examine issues such as rapid sharing of information and generic medicines.

World Health Organization

The WHO's international collaborative programme on drug safety was originally set up in 1968 and since 1978 the Uppsala Monitoring Centre (UMC) in Sweden has provided scientific leadership and technical support to this expanding worldwide pharmacovigilance network.

The WHO programme began with only a handful of participating countries but, by 2016, the number of countries included had risen to 153 (124 full members and 29 associate members). Some national centres with particular pharmacovigilance expertise have become WHO Collaborating Centres. More recently established Collaborating Centres include Ghana (2009), Morocco (2012) and Lareb in the Netherlands, which provides additional expertise in the areas of patient reporting and pharmacovigilance curriculum development. The main WHO-UMC programme activities of today are as follows:

1) *Programme for International Drug Monitoring (PIDM)*   All countries that are members of the WHO-PIDM provide their post-marketing individual case safety reports to the UMC, where the data are entered into the global reference source, VigiBase. By December 2015, there were over 12 million reports in VigiBase, accessible to all national pharmacovigilance centres through UMC's web-based search and analysis tool, VigiLyze. Data requests can also be made by anyone with a legitimate interest in the reports contained in VigiBase, although charges may be levied on those outside national centres.

2) *Training and support for participating countries*   The UMC and its Collaborating Centres offer training and support to any country wishing to set up and develop a national pharmacovigilance centre. Examples of newly established centres since 2000 include Sri Lanka (2000), Ghana (2001), Peru (2002), Sudan (2008), Jamaica (2012) and Swaziland (2015); a full list can be found on the UMC website (Box 6.1). Many countries – especially developing nations – start with little resource, few staff and a low number of reports submitted, but once in the WHO programme many develop into larger and more productive centres. In addition to on-the-ground support, regular training and education sessions are provided to WHO programme members, and there is also an annual WHO National Centres meeting which is held at different locations around the world. Some of these annual meetings are timed to run back-to-back with the annual ISoP conference, with joint sessions on an overlapping day to encourage greater international collaboration.

3) *Providing products and commercial services*   More than 70 WHO programme members use the web-based data management

---

Box 6.1 Key website references.

Council for International Organizations of Medical Sciences: www.cioms.ch

Drug Information Association: www.diaglobal.org

International Council on Harmonisation: http://www.ich.org/home.html

International Society of Pharmacoepidemiology: www.pharmacoepi.org

International Society of Pharmacovigilance: http://isoponline.org/about-isop/

United States Food and Drug Administration Sentinel Initiative: http://www.fda.gov/Safety/FDAsSentinelInitiative/ucm149340.htm

World Health Organization Uppsala Monitoring Centre: www.who-umc.org

---

system, VigiFlow, developed by the UMC. Commercial services offered by the UMC include the WHO Drug Dictionary Enhanced, which is offered mainly to industry and research organisations. The UMC no longer provides subscriptions to the WHO Adverse Reaction Terminology (WHO-ART), but continues to provide the WHO-ART to MedDRA Bridge, which is intended to help countries migrate to MedDRA (see Glossary).

4) *Pharmacovigilance analysis and research* For signal detection and investigation, the UMC uses a data-mining approach (see Chapter 4) supported by additional triage algorithms, and clinical assessment provided by UMC experts and a panel of reviewers. The UMC's research department undertakes methodology research, including data mining of electronic healthcare records and structured benefit–risk assessment.

5) *Communicating drug safety information worldwide* Information is exchanged within the WHO programme network through the publication of the *WHO Pharmaceuticals Newsletter*, and electronically through the VigiMed collaboration portal. The UMC distributes the *Signal* document, containing summaries of signals recently investigated, and publishes *Uppsala Reports*, a magazine giving information on current pharmacovigilance topics and news from centres around the world.

Council for International Organizations of Medical Sciences

The CIOMS is an international, non-profit, non-governmental organisation established jointly by the WHO and United Nations Educational, Scientific and Cultural Organization (UNESCO) in 1949. It has served as a forum for discussions between regulators and industry on a variety of pharmacovigilance topics since the late 1980s and reports from CIOMS working groups have been highly influential in shaping legislation and guidelines around the world. In 2013, membership of the CIOMS included 49 international and associate member organisations.

The activities of CIOMS can be broadly divided into three areas:

1) Drug development research
2) Human ethics, particularly in medical research
3) Working groups to produce guidance on drug safety issues.

Here, we focus on the CIOMS working groups as these have the most direct relevance to pharmacovigilance. Between 1990 and 2015 10 formal CIOMS working groups have been established, the topics and broad vision of each are summarised next.

CIOMS I: International Reporting of ADRs (1990)

Before the mid-1980s, reporting requirements to regulatory authorities related almost entirely to ADR reports occurring on each national territory. Some countries then started to introduce requirements for submission of 'foreign' reports. This working group was convened to discuss the principles of what should be reported and how. The key output was that 'foreign' reports should be of suspected reactions which were both serious *and* unexpected (i.e. unlabelled) and should be submitted within 15 days.

This CIOMS group also developed a reporting form – the 'CIOMS form' – which became the international standard. In 1995, the working group reconvened (as CIOMS Ia) and made proposals for the data elements to be included in electronic transmission of reports. Today, this form, known as the CIOMS 1 form, is still used for ADR reporting, although the current international standard for reporting is now the ICH E2B format, which was developed based on the data elements described in CIOMS Ia.

CIOMS II: International Reporting of Periodic Safety Update Summaries (1992)

This report made the original proposals for the format and content of Periodic Safety Update Reports (PSURs). Since 1992, requirements for PSURs have been widely implemented as a regulatory requirement and there is now a European GVP Module covering this subject (see Chapter 5). A harmonised guideline has also been adopted through the ICH.

CIOMS III: Guidelines for Preparing Core Clinical-Safety Information on Drugs (1995)

The third CIOMS report addressed the problem of variations in safety labelling around the world by proposing that manufacturers should develop 'core clinical-safety information' which contains all the relevant safety information that needs to be included in all countries where the drug is marketed. This is effectively a minimum standard – additional information may be included in some countries – and it also serves as the basis for deciding whether a specific adverse reaction is 'listed' (i.e. expected).

CIOMS IV: Benefit–Risk Balance for Marketed Drugs – Evaluating Safety Signals (1998)

This report proposed a standard format and content for a benefit–risk evaluation report and also laid down the principles for good decision-making practices. The CIOMS IV working group recommended a harmonised approach to the analysis, reporting and decision-making steps involved in any re-evaluation of benefit–risk that is required when safety issues arise.

CIOMS V: Current Challenges in Pharmacovigilance – Pragmatic Approaches (2001)

CIOMS V covered good case management and reporting practices, both in terms of individual cases and summaries. It included specific recommendations and was intended to be used as a handbook in pharmacovigilance departments. A general recommendation was that the ultimate goal should be a single, global, shared dataset.

CIOMS VI: Management of Safety Information from Clinical Trials (2005)

The aim of this report was to enhance awareness of the ethical and technical issues associated with safety in clinical trials. The working group proposed a systematic approach to managing safety during clinical development. The CIOMS VI report was wide ranging, covering ethical issues, statistical approaches to identifying risks and communication of safety information from clinical trials.

CIOMS VII: The Development Safety Update Report – Harmonising the Format and Content for Periodic Safety Reporting During Clinical Trials (2006)

This report proposed the content and format for a Development Safety Update Report (DSUR), a means of regular and timely review, appraisal and communication of safety information during the clinical development of drugs. The working group suggested that the DSUR and PSUR could be integrated into a single harmonised safety report that would cover a product throughout its life cycle.

CIOMS VIII: Practical Aspects of Signal Detection in Pharmacovigilance (2010)

This working group looked at how electronic capture of data was resulting in the accrual of large datasets with much potential for complex analyses. The CIOMS VIII report gave practical recommendations for how such datasets could be managed for signal detection and how pharmacovigilance systems and practices could be strengthened.

CIOMS IX: Practical Approaches to Risk Minimisation for Medicinal Products (2014)

The CIOMS Working Group IX was set up in 2010 to develop a pragmatic consensus publication that would contain a harmonised list of tools for managing the risks of medicinal products, as well as considerations governing the potential application of these tools. Following review, drafting and wider consultation, the group's report was published in 2014.

CIOMS X: Meta-analysis

The 10th CIOMS working group was set up to consider how good meta-analysis practices could be applied to clinical safety data within the biopharmaceutical regulatory process. Meta-analyses (see Chapter 3) have been increasingly used to examine risks and benefits of medicines and there is continuing debate as to the value of this approach. The report from this working group was expected to be published during 2016.

Other Activities of CIOMS

In addition to the projects discussed, CIOMS working groups have also addressed the following issues:

- Vaccine pharmacovigilance
- Pharmacogenetics
- Drug development research and pharmacovigilance in resource-poor countries.

CIOMS has also been involved in developing definitions of ADR terms and, in particular, definitions for the frequencies at which ADRs are reported to occur (see Chapter 4).

International Council on Harmonisation

Formerly known as the International Conference on Harmonisation, which was established in 1990, the organisation was renamed the International Council for Harmonisation of Technical Requirements for Pharmaceuticals for Human Use (ICH) in 2015. The aim of the ICH is to bring together regulatory authorities and the pharmaceutical industry to discuss scientific and technical aspects of drug registration. It is a more formal group than CIOMS, which is more an ideas 'think tank' which produces reports, and has a wider remit for harmonisation across the drug development process.

The ICH has also been influential in shaping current regulatory requirements relating to pharmacovigilance, particularly through its guidance documents. It was previously tripartite in terms of regions, covering the EU, the USA/Canada and Japan, but is now open to any country fulfilling the requirements set out in the ICH Articles of Association. In addition to representatives from regulation and industry, there are various observers including the WHO and International Federation of Pharmaceutical Manufacturers and Associations. The main purpose is to harmonise existing guidelines related to development and registration of medicines.

ICH guidelines have a five-step development process:

- Step 1 – Preliminary discussion by relevant experts and production of a draft
- Step 2 – The draft is considered and signed-off by the Management Committee
- Step 3 – Wider consultation and revision
- Step 4 – Final sign-off by the Management Committee
- Step 5 – Implementation into the relevant legislation and guidelines.

In principle, the authorities in each territory are committed to implementing ICH guidelines, although in practice the timing and extent of implementation have been variable.

There are four broad categories of ICH guideline:

1) *Quality* – for example, guidelines on the conduct of stability studies.
2) *Safety* – covering *pre-clinical* risks such as genotoxicity, reproductive toxicity and carcinogenicity. A notable ICH safety guideline examined non-clinical testing to assess the risk of QT prolongation with certain medicines.
3) *Efficacy* – these guidelines cover the design, conduct, *safety* (note that ICH includes pharmacovigilance in the 'Efficacy' guidelines group) and reporting of clinical trials.
4) *Multi-disciplinary* – these cover topics that do not fit neatly into any of the above three categories – for example, the ICH medical terminology (MedDRA), the Common Technical Document (CTD) and the development of Electronic Standards for the Transfer of Regulatory Information (ESTRI).

In relation to pharmacovigilance, the key ICH guidelines are E2A-E2F (included in the Efficacy group above) and the dates at which they were implemented were as follows:

- E2A: Definitions and Standards for Expedited Reporting (1994)
- E2B: Data Elements for Electronic transmission of Individual Case Safety Reports (1997)
- E2C: Periodic Safety Update Reports for Marketed Drugs (1996)
- E2D: Post-approval Safety Data Management (2003)
- E2E: Pharmacovigilance Planning (2005)
- E2F: Development Safety Update Report (2010).

ICH guideline E2E had a significant international impact, its key message being that additional methods to spontaneous reporting are required to monitor the safety of medicines adequately in the post-marketing period. In the years that followed publication of E2E, the US FDA developed the Sentinel Initiative for additional monitoring of medicines and the EU worked towards introducing more regulatory requirements for risk management planning (see Chapter 5).

International Scientific Collaboration

Earlier chapters of this book discuss basic methods and tools for pharmacovigilance (see Chapter 2) and the types and sources of data that are used in the scientific investigation of drug safety issues (see Chapter 3). It is worth noting here that the science and methodology of pharmacovigilance has developed substantially in recent years, and that much of this has been a result of international collaborative efforts. In addition to the work carried out by regulatory bodies and the international organisations, a significant amount of pharmacovigilance and pharmacoepidemiology research has been performed by academic institutions around the world. Many studies have been international multi-centre studies, especially investigations of less common outcomes, where large numbers of patients need to be included to obtain meaningful results. Researchers, academics and clinicians worldwide have collaborated with national pharmacovigilance centres, WHO collaborating centres and other non-governmental organisations to develop scientifically robust methods for the practice of pharmacovigilance (see Chapter 4).

International Professional Societies

Much international collaboration in pharmacovigilance occurs through professional societies which support their members in encouraging sharing of information and ideas and promoting research. Collegial networking in these societies is valued by those working in the different areas where pharmacovigilance is practiced (e.g. regulation, industry, academia/research, clinical work) and over many years has resulted in numerous professional collaborations.

There are several professional bodies for people working in pharmacovigilance and some are based on the members' qualifications (e.g. pharmacists' associations in different countries) or their employment role (e.g. the Regulatory Affairs Professionals Society). There are three broader international professional societies, which do not require specific qualifications or employment roles for membership, as follows.

International Society of Pharmacovigilance (ISoP)

IsoP began in 1993 as the European Society of Pharmacovigilance (ESoP) and for the first few years activities and meetings were mainly for those working in Europe. However, in 2001, ESoP became ISoP and there has since been a strong focus on increasing the international reach of the society. There are now several regional chapters of ISoP including the Western Pacific, Latin American, Middle Eastern and African chapters, in addition to several European chapters.

ISoP organises an annual research-based conference (held alternate years in Europe and outside Europe) and also offers training courses for members throughout the year. Abstracts from ISoP conferences are published in the international journal *Drug Safety*. ISoP also runs several special interest groups (SIGs) including Risk Communication and Women's Medicines. It describes itself as a society that is 'professional, independent, non-profit and open to anyone with an interest in the safety and effectiveness of medicines'.

International Society for Pharmacoepidemiology (ISPE)

ISPE began in 1989 as a North American and European society and includes those working in the broader field of pharmacoepidemiology in addition to pharmacovigilance. Like ISoP, ISPE has become more international in recent years and has regional chapters. It also now holds an annual pharmacoepidemiology conference in Asia, in addition to its other meetings. Abstracts from ISPE meetings are published in the international journal *Pharmacoepidemiology and Drug Safety*.

ISPE also has several SIGs, including those covering drug utilisation research, medical devices and vaccines. It is a larger society than ISoP and there is some collaboration and networking between the two societies. Both ISoP and ISPE have links with CIOMS and ICH, and many working in pharmacovigilance worldwide are members of more than one group.

Drug Information Association

The Drug Information Association (DIA) was founded in 1964 as a 'neutral global membership association' which aimed to provide a forum for all those working in healthcare product development (especially in industry and regulation) to discuss pertinent issues. Its goals of communication and collaboration in the area of drug development remain the same and issues relating to safety of medicines and benefit assessment still fall under the DIA umbrella. However, members of DIA are more likely to be those working in pre-licensing drug development, rather than post-marketing pharmacovigilance and pharmacoepidemiology.

Conclusions

Pharmacovigilance is an international activity and collaboration and communication are needed more than ever before to monitor the safety of products marketed worldwide. Much pharmacovigilance and pharmacoepidemiology research and monitoring is conducted all around the world. While the USA and Europe continue to play a major part in regulation, research and development, other countries outside these regions have much to contribute in the area of post-marketing surveillance.

There is a continuing need for practical pharmacovigilance in *all* countries where medicines are marketed, and the WHO worldwide pharmacovigilance programme includes over 150 countries. Other international bodies, including the CIOMS and ICH, have made significant contributions to pharmacovigilance guidance and continue to provide forums for international discussions. Three international professional societies – ISoP, ISPE and the DIA – also provide members with opportunities for communication, discussion of research and collaboration across the world.

7

Clinical Aspects of Adverse Drug Reactions

In clinical practice, prescription of a medicine is the most common intervention. Prescribing rates have increased in many countries in recent years: in England, the number of prescriptions dispensed increased between 2006 and 2013 from approximately 15 to 19 per person per year. In 2013, over 1 billion items were prescribed in England alone, costing £8.63 billion during that year. The monetary costs of prescribing such large numbers of medicines are only one aspect of the impact of this frequent clinical intervention. Equally significant are the consequences for patient safety. A report by the American Institute of Medicine, 'To Err is Human', identified adverse drug reactions (ADRs) as the most common clinical adverse event. In the UK, which has a population of around 60 million, the total number of spontaneously reported ADRs has increased in recent years. In 2015, a total of 39 046 reports were received by the MHRA compared to 21 419 in 2006. In everyday practice, side effects to medicines result in high mortality and morbidity rates and cause much clinical burden.

Pharmacovigilance has its roots in clinical practice – this is where the majority of ADR reports originate – and the most important aim of all pharmacovigilance activities should be to improve patient safety in every clinical setting. People take medicines in a wide variety of environments, most often in the community where they live, but also in hospitals and other care facilities, in schools, residential homes and prisons. Others volunteer to take medicines as part of a clinical trial or research study, either as healthy participants or for a specific condition. It is important to understand the clinical context in which medicines are used and how medicines have many benefits. Some

An Introduction to Pharmacovigilance, Second Edition. Patrick Waller and Mira Harrison-Woolrych.

treatments have completely changed the prognosis or quality of life for patients; for example, statins for the primary and secondary prevention of cardiovascular disease and isotretinoin for the treatment of severe acne. However, all medicines have side effects and in earlier chapters we have discussed benefit–risk evaluation in the processes and practice of pharmacovigilance. Nowhere is this assessment more important than in the clinical setting, where health professionals need to communicate the potential benefits and harms of medicines directly to patients and their caregivers.

In this chapter we give an overview of the clinical aspects of adverse drug events and some examples of important ADRs encountered in medical practice. We then consider some specific patient populations and discuss how patient safety could be improved in the clinical environment.

Clinical Burden of ADRs

ADRs are an important cause of morbidity and mortality in many clinical settings and continue to place a major demand on public health services worldwide. In 2004, a British study reported that 6.5% of hospital admissions were directly a result of an ADR, with a projected annual cost to the National Health Service of £466 million. A systematic review which included 25 observational studies (with a total of more than 100 000 patients) reported that about 5% of hospital admissions were associated with an adverse drug event. Thus, the burden of ADRs on hospital systems – and the associated costs – is significant.

Data on the prevalence of ADRs in patients in the community are more difficult to find. A prospective cohort study of over 1200 patients attending four primary care practices in Boston, USA, found that about one-quarter of people who responded to the survey experienced an adverse drug event and about 13% of all events identified were classified as serious. The effects of ADRs on patients (and healthcare professionals and systems) in general practice can be wide-reaching. In addition to the mortality and morbidity directly caused by ADRs, there may be indirect clinical effects; for example, issues affecting medication adherence. A patient experiencing clinically significant adverse events related to a medicine (e.g. gastro-intestinal effects caused by metformin prescribed for diabetes) may be less compliant and even stop taking the medicine completely. In the example of a patient prescribed metformin this may lead to poor blood glucose control and worsening diabetes, with more clinical consequences.

ADRs are an important form of iatrogenic (i.e. doctor-induced) disease. Many of the serious reactions that occur are well-recognised and potentially preventable; for example, bleeding with warfarin, or the upper gastro-intestinal effects of non-steroidal anti-inflammatory drugs (NSAIDs). In public health terms, it is not newly introduced drugs that are responsible for most of the population effects of adverse drugs reactions, but those whose safety profile is 'well-established'.

The burden of ADRs on people's lives can extend far outside the clinical environments in which they are treated. There are many less measurable impacts of illness; for example, dependency on family or other carers, lost working hours (and hence financial cost), time away from education or training opportunities and reduced quality of life. For older patients – a group at high risk of ADRs – the last point is especially important. It could be argued that there is little point prescribing medicines to extend the number of years of life if those years are of such poor quality that they cannot be enjoyed.

Important ADRs and Minimising Risk

The most important ADRs in clinical practice are those that cause serious morbidity and mortality – that is, those that are potentially life-threatening. There are many examples of such ADRs – from general anaphylaxis to serious adverse events affecting any body system. It is beyond the scope of this book to describe them all and so instead we have chosen some examples of important ADRs and discuss how the risks of these serious events can be minimised in clinical practice.

Gastro-intestinal Bleeding

Bleeding from the gastro-intestinal tract is a recognised side effect of some of the most commonly prescribed medicines, including NSAIDs, selective serotonin re-uptake inhibitors (SSRIs), warfarin and the newer novel oral anticoagulants (NOACs), alendronate and other bisphosphonate medicines, and corticosteroids such as prednisolone (or prednisone in the USA and Oceania). Long-term users of NSAIDs (e.g. patients with arthritis, other inflammatory conditions or chronic pain) have a 1–4% annual risk of gastro-intestinal bleeding and it has been estimated in the UK that this causes 12 000 emergency admissions and 2200 deaths per year.

Gastro-intestinal bleeding can occur from any region of the tract – from the mouth, teeth and gums down to the rectum and anus – and may range from relatively minor, to major life-threatening haemorrhage. Commonly affected areas are the stomach and small intestine, where gastro-intestinal bleeding may present as haematemesis (vomiting blood). Gastro-intestinal haemorrhage may also present as melaena (dark stools) or rectal bleeding. Patients most at risk include the elderly, those taking anticoagulants, patients with pre-existing disorders of coagulation and those on multiple medicines, especially other medicines known to cause gastro-intestinal bleeding.

The pharmaceutical industry has attempted to reduce the risk of gastro-intestinal bleeding associated with many medicines by developing new products; for example, enteric-coated NSAIDs, more selective cyclo-oxygenase 2 (COX-2) inhibitors and combination products (e.g. tablets containing a NSAID and a prostaglandin), and some of these have been successful. Other ways of minimising the risk of drug-related gastro-intestinal bleeding in clinical practice include the following:

- Identifying patients at high risk by taking a thorough family history, reviewing all clinical details for each patient including a full medication history, including herbals and other over-the-counter (OTC) medicines such as aspirin, and alcohol intake.
- Reducing drug use in high-risk patients, for example older people.
- Prescribing the lowest possible dose for the shortest possible time period.
- Prescribing the medicine with the lowest risk; for example, ibuprofen as the NSAID with the lowest risk of gastro-intestinal bleeding.
- Consider co-prescribing acid secretion blocking medicines.
- Informing patients of the risk of gastro-intestinal bleeding and encouraging them to present early to medical services if such side effects occur (this is important for reducing fatalities).

Agranulocytosis and Other Blood Dyscrasias

Some medicines have adverse effects on blood cells, including granulocytes (white blood cells) which are a vital component of the immune system. An example of a medicine that can affect the number of neutrophils (the most common type of granulocyte) is clozapine, an atypical antipsychotic prescribed for treatment-resistant schizophrenia. Clozapine has an important place in clinical practice as it is very effective in some patients who do not respond to other antipsychotic medicines, or who have specific symptoms which are difficult to control with other medicines. It has been reported that approximately 30–60% of patients with schizophrenia resistant to other treatments will respond to clozapine.

While clozapine is clinically effective in a group of patients who have limited other options, it is also associated with serious side effects including myocarditis (inflammation of the heart muscle), gastro-intestinal dysmotility (causing severe constipation in some patients) and serious haematological effects. The frequency of neutropenia (defined in most countries as a neutrophil count of less than 1.5×10^9/L) in clozapine-treated patients is 2% and of agranulocytosis (defined as a neutrophil count of less than 0.5×10^9/L) is 0.8%. Agranulocytosis may be life-threatening, or even fatal, as the patient's immune system is severely compromised.

For some medicines, identification of such a serious ADR – with associated deaths reported –have resulted in permanent withdrawal from the market if the risks were thought to outweigh the benefits of treatment. However, the importance of clozapine in clinical practice was recognised and pharmaceutical companies – working in collaboration with clinicians, researchers and regulators – developed a risk-minimisation solution which allowed clozapine to be authorised for schizophrenia resistant to other treatments. In several countries, clozapine manufacturers have developed mandatory monitoring programmes in which patients' blood samples are regularly tested to detect haematological adverse effects.

In clinical practice, clozapine is started by the patient's psychiatrist and should only be prescribed if the patient has not responded to other antipsychotic medications. Blood tests are performed before clozapine is started (a normal white cell count is required) and then at least weekly for the first 18 weeks of treatment. After that time, blood tests are required at 2-week intervals during the first year and then at

4-week intervals for the remainder of the time on treatment (and also for 4 weeks after stopping treatment). Pharmacists have an important role in clozapine risk management programmes, as they check that blood tests have been performed before dispensing the patient's next dose of clozapine. Some schemes have a 'red, amber, green' approach to guide prescribers and pharmacists, with a 'red' result indicating that clozapine should not be prescribed if white cell counts have fallen too low. Community psychiatric nurses also play an important part in supporting patients on clozapine.

Common Clinical Scenarios

These examples outline how potentially serious ADRs can be managed effectively in clinical practice and how life-threatening outcomes can be prevented, but there are many other examples in everyday practice where management of patients is not as clear-cut. In Box 7.1 we describe a common clinical case scenario involving management of a patient concerned about side effects from statins.

This case reveals some of the complexities of identifying and managing ADRs in real-life clinical practice. Muscle aches and worsening memory are both common complaints in older patients and there may be other factors (e.g. increased physical activity) that may be responsible for the onset of new symptoms. It is also possible that new symptoms represent new-onset disease (e.g. polymyalgia rheumatica or polymyositis) rather than an ADR. Physical examination and blood tests help the doctor exclude or confirm certain conditions, but as seen in the case history, often there is not a specific blood test for a particular symptom or ADR and results can be equivocal rather than giving an exact diagnosis. In this case, the positive dechallenge and rechallenge suggested that the patient's muscle symptoms were likely caused by the first statin, but in practice it is not always easy to get such evidence – for example, if a patient is unwilling to restart a medicine that caused them to have unpleasant symptoms. Finally, in the case in Box 7.1, changing to another statin helped the patient's muscle symptoms (while theoretically myalgia is a class effect of statins, in practice many patients find they do not get symptoms with another medicine of the same class) but did not give as effective control of her blood lipids. This shows that in real life, often a compromise position has to be reached.

Box 7.1 Case history.

Mrs X, a 61-year-old woman, visits her GP for a review of her statin medication and a repeat prescription. A year earlier, she had been invited to have a cardiovascular risk assessment with the practice nurse and was found to have hyperlipidaemia (increased levels of fats in the blood) which gave her an elevated cardiovascular risk score. She was advised to make dietary changes, but these did not significantly alter her cholesterol ratio, so Mrs X was commenced on a statin medication (HMG-CoA reductase inhibitor).

At her medication review, Mrs X mentions to her GP that she has read on the internet about 'muscle problems' and memory loss with statins. She feels her memory has deteriorated in the past year and that she has been experiencing more general aches and pains. Mrs X asks her GP if these symptoms could be caused by the statin. On further discussion, she also reports that she has recently retired, has been redecorating her house and has been much more active in her garden. Her GP checks that she is not on any other concomitant medications, including herbal treatments and over-the-counter products.

The GP examines Mrs X and finds no evidence of muscle tenderness or weakness. Blood tests are performed for creatine kinase (an enzyme marker of muscle breakdown) and serum cholesterol. A few days later Mrs X is told her tests show her cholesterol levels are under good control on the present dosage of statin. Although her creatine kinase is slightly raised, it is not enough to indicate rhabdomyolysis (muscle breakdown) or myositis (muscle inflammation). Mrs X is still concerned about her symptoms and so it is agreed that she will stop the statin for 2 weeks (dechallenge) to see if her symptoms improve and then restart the medicine at the same dose (rechallenge).

After stopping the statin, Mrs X notices a marked improvement in her muscle pains, but no change in her memory. On restarting the medicine, her muscle pain returns (positive rechallenge) so her GP advises trying a lower dose. Mrs X reduces the dosage but still experiences muscle symptoms and after further discussion her GP switches her to another statin. She tolerates this drug without muscle side effects, but her blood lipids are not as well controlled as with the first statin. Mrs X is unwilling to try a higher dosage of the new statin, so it is agreed she will remain on this dosage and accept the risks of less tightly controlled hyperlipidaemia.

Other common clinical scenarios are less complicated – for example, a patient who presents with a drug rash, which is easily identified through taking a clear history and clinical examination. Skin ADRs are among the most commonly reported group of reactions reported to regulatory authorities and fall into several groups:

- Erythematous (redness), maculo-papular (flat and raised redness) or exanthematous (blotchy redness)
- Urticarial (sometimes known as hives or nettle rash)
- Angioedema (swelling of the face, lips, oral cavity and upper respiratory tract)
- Photosensitivity (skin reaction to sunlight)
- Purpuric (bruising or bleeding under the skin)
- Fixed drug eruption (recurrence at same site)
- Bullous (blistering) conditions (e.g. bullous pemphigoid or sub-epidermal blistering)
- Widespread skin reactions (e.g. Stevens–Johnson syndrome, SJS; toxic epidermal necrolysis, TEN).

Most skin ADRs are not serious and resolve on cessation of the medicine and symptomatic treatment, but some require biopsy by a specialist. However, some skin reactions are very serious – for example, SJS or TEN (Figure 7.1) – and can affect the whole body. Such reactions are life-threatening and require intensive treatment, despite which they are sometimes fatal.

Important Patient Populations

While it is important to remember that any patient can experience an ADR to any medicine at any time (not all ADRs occur in the first days or weeks of treatment), some patients are at higher risk of ADRs:

- *Women* – in every age group, women take more medicines than men (including contraceptive products, herbals and OTC medicines), may metabolise medicines differently and experience more ADRs. In the UK, in 2015, more spontaneous ADR reports were received for women (56%) than men (39%), with gender unspecified in some cases.
- *Older patients* – the elderly are prescribed more medicines than younger patients, take medicines for longer periods, have more

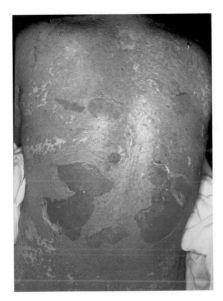

Figure 7.1 Photograph of patient with toxic epidermal necrolysis (TEN).
© DermNet New Zealand. We are grateful to DermNet New Zealand for
permission to reproduce the image under the terms of this license:
https://creativecommons.org/licenses/by-nc-nd/3.0/nz/legalcode.

pre-existing disease (including deteriorating hepatic and renal
function) giving more chance of ADRs and drug interactions.
Recent UK data show that the age band with the highest number of
spontaneous ADR reports per year was 61–70 years (note that these
are absolute numbers of reports and not frequencies of ADRs).

- *Patients with chronic (long-term) conditions* – examples include
those with diabetes, autoimmune conditions, epilepsy, arthritis or
other joint conditions, schizophrenia and other chronic psychoses,
hypertension, heart disease, and chronic lung disease. These
patients are likely to be on long-term medications, may be taking
several medicines and there may also be aspects of their conditions
that make them more susceptible to ADRs.

- *Patients with genetic or other susceptibilities affecting how medicines
are metabolised* – for example glucose-6-phospate dehydrogenate
deficiency (an X-linked recessive enzyme deficiency which affects
about 400 million people worldwide) which alters metabolism of
several medicines including antibiotics and antimalarials.

In addition to the above groups, there are special populations where exposure to medicines should be carefully considered, as follows.

Pregnant Women

Virtually all medicines cross the placenta, resulting in fetal exposure, so it is important for clinicians and women to consider this risk, especially as many pregnancies are unplanned. However, it is also important to remember that some women require medicines during pregnancy, for example those with epilepsy or other chronic conditions. The benefit–risk assessment of medicines in pregnancy may be quite complex and it advisable to refer to specialist sources of information (see Chapter 10).

Breastfeeding Infants and Neonates

Babies may be exposed to medicines via their mothers' milk and it is important for clinicians to take a maternal drug history – including herbals, OTC medicines and alcohol. Neonates can be at more risk of ADRs because of their immature metabolic systems and dose adjustment of medicines is crucial in this very young population, especially for premature babies.

Children

While the number of medicines licensed for use in the paediatric population is increasing all the time, it may still be necessary for clinicians to prescribe medicines to children 'off-label' (i.e. outside the terms of the marketing authorisation). Data are often lacking in patients under 18 years and, as for neonates, dosage adjustments may have to be made in small children. Younger people may also be at risk of specific ADRs (e.g. Reye's syndrome with aspirin).

Improving Patient Safety in Clinical Practice

We began this chapter by placing pharmacovigilance at the centre of patient safety, not least because ADRs are the most common safety event in clinical practice, both in community and hospital settings. Patient safety is the ultimate goal of all pharmacovigilance practice and in everyday clinical practice there are several steps that can be taken to improve this outcome.

Better Prescribing

To reduce the clinical burden of ADRs, prescribers should discuss four important questions with patients before reaching for the prescription pad:

1) *Is this medicine really needed?* There may be non-pharmaceutical alternatives which should be tried first – for example, dietary changes and exercise programmes before weight reduction medicines are prescribed.
2) *Is this medicine suitable for this person and this condition?* For example, antidepressant medicines are not usually an appropriate treatment for grief.
3) *How effective is this medicine likely to be?* It is generally not well understood by patients that most medicines are *not* 100% effective – many products are only effective in around 50% of patients. This is an important consideration for benefit–risk discussions in the clinical setting.
4) *How safe is this medicine?* What are the most common and most serious ADRs associated with the medicine? Is the patient in a high-risk group or in a special population requiring extra consideration? Most people understand that all drugs have some side effects, but may not understand that some of these may be life-threatening.

Avoiding Medication Error

In all clinical settings, steps can be taken to reduce medication error, which has been defined as 'a failure in the treatment process that leads to, or has the potential to lead to, harm to the patient' and includes different types of error, for example prescription of the wrong drug or giving an incorrect dose. Protocols may involve several different members of a multi-disciplinary team, for example doctors, nurses and pharmacists each making checks during the process of prescribing and dispensing a medicine. In many countries, prevention of medication errors is now part of pharmacovigilance practice and adverse events should be reported to national systems.

An important point is that these adverse events should be entirely preventable with good clinical practice.

Use of Available Guidance

For many drugs or conditions (e.g. disease-modifying anti-rheumatoid drugs for rheumatological conditions) there are guidance documents, checklists and treatment/monitoring protocols available to clinicians. These are drawn up by international, national or more local authorities. Using and adhering to such guidance has potential to reduce ADRs and/or detect ADRs early in order to reduce harm to patients on long-term medicines.

Medication Reviews

For patients taking medicines in the long term, it is helpful for clinicians – ideally in collaboration with pharmacists and other members of the patient's healthcare team – to undertake regular medication reviews. This is especially important in the elderly population or other groups at high risk of ADRs. It is fairly common for additional medicines to be prescribed to older patients presenting with new problems, without considering whether any other medicines could be discontinued. Regular medication review, involving the patient and their carers, has much potential to improve patient safety and quality of life.

Good Communication

As in all other areas of pharmacovigilance practice (see Chapter 4), good communication is essential in the clinical setting. Clear explanations and discussions which consider the patient's perspective are at the heart of the clinical consultation. Use of diagrams, pictures and charts can help explain risks of medicines in lay language. There are also many useful resources to support the patient after the consultation – in particular, the product's *Patient Information Leaflet (PIL)* which should be provided to the patient when the medicine is dispensed. In most countries, the product's PIL (known as the *package leaflet* in the EU, *package insert* in the USA and *consumer information leaflet* in some other regions) is assessed as part of the regulatory process, to check it complies with the licensed product information in accurately describing ADRs and other safety information, and is also readable and useful to patients and their carers. There are many other leaflets and online resources available for specific patient groups, or for specific medicines, but it should be noted that not all are entirely accurate (most online sites are not subject to expert review or regulation) and some may be promotional for certain products.

Vigilant Practice

Clinicians are encouraged to develop a high level of suspicion concerning evaluating clinical events which may be related to the patient's medicines. Some doctors have been defensive of the medicines they have prescribed and unwilling to acknowledge that (inadvertently) these products have harmed patients. In some countries, ADR reporting rates are thought to be low for this reason (and perhaps for other reasons, such as fear of litigation). This perspective will not improve clinical practice and patient safety in the longer term. In most countries, the mantra for reporting ADRs to national authorities is *'if in doubt, report it,'* as without reports, new signals will not be identified, clinical practice will not improve and the ultimate goal of improved patient safety will not be achieved.

Conclusions

Prescribing medicines is the most common intervention in everyday medical practice and ADRs are frequent clinical events, placing a large burden on health systems. In this chapter we have tried to give a snapshot of some clinical aspects of pharmacovigilance, with examples of important and common ADRs. Understanding how medicines are prescribed, taken and monitored in real life allows us to improve pharmacovigilance practice with the ultimate aim of improving patient safety.

8

Ethical and Societal Considerations

We now consider wider societal aspects of the safety of medicines, starting by identifying the main stakeholders and their perspectives. There is an important ethical dimension to pharmacovigilance – medicines are supposed to be beneficial and yet we know that harms will occur despite best efforts to prevent them. In the past, much information about the safety of medicines remained within companies and was only shared with regulators when required. Steps to improve transparency have been made both in terms of process and access to the relevant data, both in the pre- and post-licensing phases of drug development. Potential conflicts of interest are increasingly recognised as very important and need to be handled appropriately. Ethics committees continue to discuss the balance between benefit to society and possible harm to individuals. At times, public confidence in government systems has not been high – there has been criticism that regulators and industry are too cosy, and that patients' interests do not always come first. The media watch from a distance, waiting for something interesting to happen.

Stakeholders and Their Perspectives

The most important stakeholders in pharmacovigilance are patients who use medicines – this is, after all, why the discipline exists. Health professionals are also 'users' of the medicines they prescribe and both probably have similar expectations of the process. Broadly speaking, users of medicines expect them to have been adequately tested, to be

An Introduction to Pharmacovigilance, Second Edition. Patrick Waller and Mira Harrison-Woolrych.
© 2017 John Wiley & Sons Ltd. Published 2017 by John Wiley & Sons Ltd.

effective and 'safe' in the sense that serious harms are unlikely to occur, and to be provided with appropriate and understandable information about their use. These are in essence the goals of the regulatory process, but because of limitations that largely have a scientific basis there is a gap between expectation and reality. Patients know that side effects can occur with medicines, but generally perceive these as likely to be transient or reversible and non-serious. When a life-threatening reaction occurs with a treatment given for a relatively trivial indication, they are shocked. The prescribing doctor might be too, because he or she has unintentionally broken one of the first rules of medicine – *primum non nocere* (first, do no harm). By contrast, personnel working in drug safety, whether they are in industry, a regulator or in academia, may be unsurprised.

Patients exist not only as individuals but in groups (i.e. patient organisations) and such bodies have an important role in educating and supporting individuals who develop specific (usually chronic) diseases. Generally, patient organisations are more focused on access to treatments than on safety considerations and their perspective may well be that the need for and potential benefits of treatments outweigh quite major risks. Some patient groups are specifically based on the victims of particular treatments (e.g. there is still a prominent thalidomide action group in the UK) and they may be seeking to achieve recognition of a problem, regulatory measures against the drug or compensation for affected individuals.

Vaccines are a particularly sensitive area for understandable reasons – they are usually given to healthy individuals and often to children. One of the reasons for administering them as widely as possible may also be a benefit to society rather than the individual (i.e. 'herd' immunity). This raises an ethical dilemma if serious harms are possible. Perhaps for such reasons vaccines are unusual in that some attempts to compensate victims directly (i.e. without litigation) have been made. In most countries, society does not compensate victims of adverse drug reactions (ADRs) unless they are prepared to litigate. To win they are likely to have to prove individual causation, to demonstrate they were personally harmed by the treatment (this may be intrinsically difficult as was discussed in Chapter 2) and possibly also that the manufacturer did not take all reasonable steps to identify and prevent such harm. Litigation about medicines is a major industry in itself and extremely good business for lawyers who may actively advertise for cases (there are many such sites online) and pursue mass actions which are quite often settled out of court by companies as a means of damage limitation. Government health ministers are ultimately responsible for the overall system, but politicians generally avoid involvement – there is little in it for them but a potential minefield.

When an unexpected major drug safety issue arises, it is good copy and likely to receive a very high profile in the media. Hindsight will be liberally applied – surely this could have been predicted or avoided? – and the company and/or regulators are likely to be blamed. The plight of individual victims is highlighted, but media and public interest will generally be transient. The media see their role as to inform and entertain and vary considerably in their approach, but common to all is a focus on what they perceive will attract their customers (i.e. what 'sells newspapers'). Drug safety matters will usually do so, but some elements of the matter (e.g. uncertainties and difficult judgements) are often handled badly or ignored.

Media coverage may unnecessarily scare some people into inappropriate action (as in the Pill scares discussed in Chapter 1) but pharmacovigilance personnel should not lose sight of the potential positive power of their influence. Indeed, better handling of the media should be on their agenda. It is certainly worth sitting down with more responsible sections of the media and explaining what the problem is and discussing how they can help. Ultimately, anything that may lead to well-balanced coverage and clear, appropriate messages is worth pursuing.

In terms of trying to prevent unnecessary drug safety scares, it is worth bearing in mind recognised 'fright factors' – these are aspects of a particular risk that will tend to make most people more risk-averse. In particular, we tend to be more frightened by risks that are:

- Involuntarily taken
- Man-made
- Irreversible
- Poorly understood.

Many serious ADRs will meet all of these criteria, meaning that it is very easy for the public to become more scared than is appropriate and to lose sight of the balancing benefits. For example, following concerns that use of human insulins might mask the symptoms of hypoglycaemia in the early 1990s, some patients stopped taking insulin altogether.

All the parties mentioned are stakeholders in the process of pharmacovigilance, but usually lawyers and the media only become involved when a problem has already occurred. Industry personnel, regulators, researchers, non-governmental organisations (see Chapter 6) and individual users (i.e. patients/health professionals as discussed in Chapter 7) between them have the potential to prevent some specific problems occurring – the ultimate purpose of pharmacovigilance – whereas other stakeholders may influence the system or endeavour to promote change later in the process.

Ethical Principles

As should be clear from the discussions above, there are many potential tensions in the drug safety system – such as risk versus benefit, individual versus population good, potential therapeutic gain from innovation versus uncertainty. These are set against a background of commercial and political imperatives, the latter largely being the economics of healthcare. The need for an ethical approach and ethical safeguards is therefore manifest.

In terms of researching the safety of medicines in human subjects, there is an overarching code of ethical principles – the Declaration of Helsinki – which was originally developed under the auspices of the World Medical Association (WMA) in 1964. Since that time there have been several significant revisions to the Declaration and the current version (2013) is the only official one, replacing all earlier versions. The Declaration of Helsinki is based on principles outlined in the WMA Declaration of Geneva which binds the physician with the words, 'The health of my patient will be my first consideration', and the International Code of Medical Ethics which declares that 'A physician shall act in the patient's best interest when providing medical care.'

In the context of safety, the most important of the 37 points currently included in the Declaration of Helsinki are as follows:

- While the primary purpose of medical research is to generate new knowledge, this goal can never take precedence over the rights and interests of individual research subjects.
- All medical research involving human subjects must be preceded by careful assessment of predictable risks and burdens to the individuals and groups involved in the research in comparison with

foreseeable benefits to them and to other individuals or groups affected by the condition under investigation.

- Measures to minimise the risks must be implemented. The risks must be continuously monitored, assessed and documented by the researcher.
- Medical research involving human subjects may only be conducted if the importance of the objective outweighs the risks and burdens to the research subjects.

These have an underlying theme: *individual* patient safety is paramount. However, another key theme in the Declaration of Helsinki is consideration of the balance between the likely common good (future benefit to society) and the risk of harm to the individual when undertaking medical research. In pharmacovigilance, risk–benefit trade-offs made at the population level usually accept that some individuals will lose out. Essentially, a judgement is being made that more good than harm will occur in the population in the full knowledge that some harms cannot be prevented.

Informed Consent

When experimental research is being conducted (i.e. there is an intervention that would not occur in ordinary practice), informed consent is essential. On this point, the Declaration of Helsinki states 'Participation by individuals capable of giving informed consent as subjects in medical research must be voluntary. Although it may be appropriate to consult family members or community leaders, no individual capable of giving informed consent may be enrolled in a research study unless he or she freely agrees.' Issues become more complex when an individual is unable to give informed consent to be involved in research; for example, if they are too young, have a condition impeding their competency to consent or have died. Protocols involving these situations are usually referred to ethics committees for advice.

For non-interventional research (i.e. observational studies), consent of individuals has generally not been required and often may not be feasible, for example in large data-linkage studies. However, in today's environment of increasing importance of individual rights, most ethics committees will ask researchers to justify why informed consent should *not* be obtained for observational research. In addition to feasibility and methodological issues (e.g. if seeking consent would bias the results as people who agree to consent may differ from those who refuse) there is again the overriding ethical question of whether the common societal good overrides individual perspectives and if so, when? This is relevant, for example, to whether or not patient consent is required for ADR reporting and epidemiological research. To date, it has been generally agreed that individual consent is not required for submitting ADR reports, as this is in the common good and is also part of good clinical practice (so is not strictly 'research' although research may later be performed on the anonymised population data). However, during the clinical consultation most health professionals are likely to inform the patient they are submitting the ADR report and the individual has the right to opt out of this process if they so wish.

Privacy and Confidentiality

The patient's right to privacy is a key issue and individual patient data need to be held securely and treated with respect. Research protocols need to specify measures for keeping individual data private and confidential during studies and these principles also apply in post-marketing pharmacovigilance practice. Often it is necessary to de-identify personal data for research purposes and no individual should be identifiable when results are shared with authorities or published. While there is a general statement about privacy and confidentiality in the Declaration of Helsinki, it should be noted that legislation varies considerably between countries and this needs to be considered when performing international pharmacoepidemiology research.

Ethical Issues for the Pharmaceutical Industry

There are various other specific ethical issues that face industry personnel and are relevant to safety. For example:

- Ethical promotion of drugs, given the potential link between safety and promotion.
- Public representation of data (e.g. the temptation towards suppression of unfavourable data or expert opinions).

- Drug pricing and availability, especially in the developing world, may lead to use of less safe medicines.
- Control over publication of results that were unfavourable in terms of efficacy or safety.

Ethical Safeguards in Relation to Safety

The safeguards in place to protect patient safety can broadly be considered on the following four levels.

Legislation, Voluntary Codes and Guidelines

Many of the issues discussed are addressed in the framework of medicines legislation in each country, in international codes such as the Declaration of Helsinki and ICH guidance (see Chapter 6) and in national and regional ethical guidelines. The pharmaceutical industry also has some voluntary codes (e.g. in relation to advertising practices), as do health professionals, whose professional bodies have developed codes and guidelines for ethical practice.

Ethics Committees/Review Boards

Ethics committees operate nationally or regionally and the role of such committees is to consider ethical aspects of specific research proposals. Committee membership is usually comprised of both expert (medical or scientific) and lay representatives and in many countries meetings are open in order to increase transparency. Their key task is to protect study participants by reviewing research protocols and any amendments that may be necessary once the study is under way.

Many studies presented to ethics committee involve evaluation of the safety of medicines, either in pre-licensing clinical trials or in studies of marketed medicines. Some of the key ethical issues in such studies are as follows:

- There may be no benefit to the study participant (especially for first-in-man studies or other new indication studies) and this is an important difference to benefit–risk assessment in clinical practice.

- The risks of the medicines to be administered in the study need to be clearly stated and explained, including frequencies of ADRs (if known from previous studies) and possible outcomes for the participant.
- Any risks to special or vulnerable populations (e.g. pregnant women, children or the elderly) need to be clearly stated and justified.
- Issues relating to participants who are unable to provide informed consent for interventional studies (e.g. unconscious patients, those with cognitive impairment).
- Researchers need to outline what they will do to minimise risk to the study participants.
- Participants must be informed of the possible risks in clear information sheets written in lay language.

Data Monitoring Committees

These should be set up for interventional studies in order to protect subjects from safety hazards which might only become evident during the course of the study. Depending on the study and the risks involved, the data monitoring committee can be an informal local group or a full external committee. These groups should be run independently of the sponsor and operate separately from those involved in the day-to-day operation of the trial. A data monitoring committee looks at the safety data sequentially as it emerges and can recommend that the trial be stopped on safety grounds if it becomes clear that patients in one treatment arm are at greater risk of a serious hazard than those in the other arm(s).

Publication

Much (but not all) medical research will eventually be published in the scientific literature. The publication process for most international journals involves peer review which thereby provides another ethical safeguard for research practice. However, publication is selective (and therefore biased) depending on:

1) *What the results show* – positive research is more likely to published than something that failed to observe a clear effect (commonly referred to as publication bias).
2) *Choices made by researchers and editors* – as with other forms of media, decisions are made regarding what is topical and of interest to readers.

Aside from the issue of non-publication (or delayed publication) of some research findings, there is also the problem of misconduct. There are many potential types of misconduct relating to publication, the most serious of which are plagiarism, fraud or fabrication. Steps have been taken to address these problems in part through the setting up of a Committee on Publication Ethics which now operates worldwide. This has drawn up guidelines intended to encourage intellectual honesty, prevent and deal with misconduct and provide advice on when research papers should be retracted.

Transparency

In the past, drug safety was, like many other processes involving regulated industry, essentially non-transparent. Users were expected to accept that behind the scenes people were doing their best and with the right motives. Commercial sensitivity was another reason given for a lack of transparency in the pharmaceutical industry. The move towards greater transparency which gained impetus during the 1990s was not specific to this field, but part of a wider societal desire to know more of what was going on. Governments have also seen advantages in opening up such processes, in terms of public confidence in systems and in increasing the credibility of their decisions and advice. This change in approach has been facilitated by developments in electronic communication. Thus, general public policy on freedom of information began to override the potential commercial considerations that were for a long time the main putative reason for secrecy. It is now generally accepted that drug safety information rarely has real commercial value to competitors.

The following is a list of some of the major types of safety data which may now be freely available:

- Published scientific literature
- Warnings on specific issues (e.g. from companies or regulatory bodies)
- Drug safety bulletins (e.g. from regulators or other professional bodies)
- Press releases
- Public assessment reports on specific issues (e.g. from regulatory bodies)

- Searchable ADR databases
- Clinical trial protocols and data.

The ordering of the list is chronological in the sense that 50 years ago only information published in the scientific literature was available and that the others have been introduced at various time points since then. The requirement for registration of clinical trials is surprisingly recent (early 2000s) and there is still scope for further development (e.g. only summaries of risk management plans have so far been made public) and in most countries, regulatory discussions are still held behind closed doors.

Timing of release of information is important because it is reasonable to be concerned that premature release before considered recommendations can be made could do more harm than good. There is also concern that complex information might be misunderstood and there is a need to improve delivery with the goal of aiding better understanding according the needs of the recipient.

Besides the information on which judgements and decisions are based, there is a need for transparency of process. In this respect the public need to know:

- Who reached the decision?
- What was the basis for the decision?
- Was the decision challenged?
- Why was another course of action not chosen?

Conflicts of Interest

The realisation that we all have conflicts of interest and attempts to deal with them is a surprisingly recent phenomenon. It was only at the beginning of the twenty-first century that one of the major journals in the field introduced a clear policy in relation to the need for declaration of such conflicts. Drug safety is now a very sensitive area in this respect because difficult judgements have to be made about the risk of serious harms and these have financial consequences for the company involved. The public need be convinced that those making the judgements are uninfluenced by such considerations and yet academic experts in the field are ubiquitously associated with, and their research is often funded by, the industry. In dealing with conflicts of interest, transparency and public credibility are the key issues.

There is general agreement that financial conflicts of interest must be disclosed and that persons with important conflicts should not influence relevant decisions. All organisations conducting pharmacovigilance work should have policies on how conflicts of interest should be handled. A useful categorisation of financial conflicts developed by regulators is to consider whether they are:

- Personal (consultancy fees, shares) or
- Non-personal (e.g. funding to a university department) and
- Specific (to the drug/issue at hand) or
- Non-specific (e.g. related to other drugs made by the same company).

Using such a system provides for four categories, and interests that are both personal and specific represent the highest level of conflict. These should result in exclusion of an expert from giving advice to regulators. Conversely, a non-personal, non-specific interest is at the lowest level and usually only requires declaration. Such systems are necessary because, in practical terms, regulators or other authorities may not have access to the necessary expertise if they simply excluded all experts who had any kind of conflict.

Other competing interests (e.g. non-financial) are also possible and systems are less well developed in dealing with them. Involvement with competitor products/companies, indirect potential conflicts via personal associations (through family or work) and past interests which might be considered lapsed, are examples of such grey areas.

Conclusions

In this chapter we have outlined broad ethical and societal considerations that impact on pharmacovigilance. We have discussed the perspectives of the relevant stakeholders and how they impact on aspects of societal behaviour when drug safety issues occur. General ethical principles and guidance are drawn from the Declaration of Helsinki and a balance is required between protecting individuals and the common good. There are some specific issues for research studies involving medicines, and ethics committees continue to be important in protecting participants from harm. To support system credibility, the need for transparency of drug safety information and processes is generally accepted, while protecting the privacy of individuals.

9

Future Directions

Current Limitations

Many new drugs have been introduced in recent decades, but there is no evidence that this has reduced the overall burden of adverse drug reactions (ADRs). Despite thorough clinical development, unexpected and sometimes unexplainable ADRs become recognised at a fairly late stage in the process. Furthermore, it is often not possible to understand why a particular individual experiences an ADR while another does not. Thus, ADRs remain an important cause of morbidity and mortality around the world (see Chapter 7). Much of this harm is potentially preventable and some of our inability to prevent it so far reflects the limitations of existing systems.

When thinking about the future of pharmacovigilance, a useful starting point is to consider the most important current limitations of the discipline. It is to be hoped that future developments will be targeted at overcoming at least some of them, although the challenges are considerable. Broadly, these limitations might be characterised under the following three headings.

1 Detecting New ADRs and Distinguishing Them from Non-causal Effects

Existing systems have many limitations for detecting new ADRs. Under-reporting is an important issue and spontaneous reporting remains a passive system, in that it relies on reporters to submit their suspicions of ADRs. More proactive methods of detecting and

An Introduction to Pharmacovigilance, Second Edition. Patrick Waller and Mira Harrison-Woolrych.
© 2017 John Wiley & Sons Ltd. Published 2017 by John Wiley & Sons Ltd.

measuring the occurrence of ADRs (e.g. prescription-event monitoring; see Chapter 3) are available but there is still not enough use of such methods and real-time monitoring has been largely focused on specific areas (e.g. vaccines).

As discussed in Chapter 2, judgement is required in deciding whether reported or observed association are causal. Such judgements are often hampered by the limitations of the available data; for example, there may not be enough clinical information provided on spontaneous reports to assess causality. Even when a causal effect appears likely, educated guesses usually have to be made about the frequency of an ADR (especially in post-marketing use) or who is most at risk and the applicability of the available data to a general population. Better use of other data sources for detecting and measuring the frequency of ADRs should also provide more detailed information on which to judge if there is direct causal relationship with the medicine.

2 Extending Knowledge of Safety

The development of risk management planning has provided a mechanism for extending knowledge of safety (i.e. gaining greater confidence that adverse effects are not remaining undetected). However, this approach is highly dependent on sponsor companies or other bodies conducting formal post-authorisation studies and remains under-utilised to date. More careful estimation of baseline risks in different groups within the population is also needed.

3 Preventing and Managing Known ADRs

Once an ADR is recognised and perhaps even well-understood, our ability to prevent it often remains imperfect for two broad reasons:

1) Few of the preventive tools used are 100% effective (e.g. monitoring liver function tests in a patient using a potentially hepatotoxic drug may only prevent some cases).
2) Most of the preventive measures available are recommendations which are imperfectly followed by clinicians and/or patients.

In overall terms, difficulties we have in predicting, understanding and measuring ADRs hamper preventive efforts, but even if those limitations could be overcome, the mechanisms for minimising known risks still need to be improved (e.g. through better communication).

Meeting the Challenges

Improving Collection of Pharmacovigilance Data

A logical approach to improving anything is to specifically target areas of weakness. For example, it is notable that one of the most toxic class of medicines, anti-cancer drugs, tend to be associated with very few ADR reports. Understanding the reasons for this (perhaps oncologists consider the side effects of these medicines are well known and therefore feel there is no need to report ADRs to regulators) may help us target and improve areas of under-reporting. In the 1990s, there was a particular difficulty in studying the then new anti-HIV drugs, which may have been related to concerns about confidentiality and the underlying diagnosis. In the UK, a targeted reporting scheme was set up which successfully allayed the concerns of reporters and gained much important information about the safety of the class.

Regarding detection of ADRs and in particular, the problem of under-reporting, such weaknesses could be overcome by the use of electronic systems at the point of prescribing. Use of reporting apps on phones are likely to allow an increased number of suspected ADR reports to be collected. The use of social media is another potential source of data for detecting ADRs, but there are several challenges with this method. It may be difficult to confirm that data refer to actual ADRs that have occurred, rather than discussion of ADRs occurring in other people (such as celebrities) or duplications of other reports. Social media may be helpful in early detection of problems in the future, but there are many aspects of this type of reporting that need further investigation.

There is also potential to improve collection of ADR data from hospital systems where, in many countries, reporting rates have been low compared with those from primary care. In the developed world, there have been hopes that electronic health record scanning could eliminate the need for spontaneous reporting as a method to detect new ADRs. However, this has proved to be difficult in practice and even developing a complete electronic record for each individual patient in a national health system has been challenging. It is to be hoped that there will be improvements in this area and the ability to test signals rapidly in large electronic systems like Sentinel in the USA is likely to improve over time. If we are successful in increasing the number of ADR reports submitted in the future, there will be a need for improvement in the methods for processing of reports and efficiently distinguishing ADRs from non-causal events.

One of the most striking areas of weakness has been in relation to children, who until recent times were largely excluded from drug development programmes and often had to be treated outside the terms of marketing authorisations (known as 'off-label' prescribing). Since 2007, this has been partially addressed through the EU regulatory requirement for *paediatric investigation plans* (with pharmacovigilance being an important element of these) and, in the UK, also by publication of a children's *British National Formulary* which gives specific advice for younger patients. While there are now more medicines licensed for paediatric use and reporting of ADRs in children has increased, there is still room for improvement.

Another area where pharmacovigilance data have been lacking is for pregnant and breastfeeding women. Again, this special population has been excluded from clinical trials and product information too often states 'no data are available'. However, some measures are being taken to improve guidance in this area, with development of a European GVP Module regarding medicines in pregnancy and lactation (see Chapter 5). In addition, healthcare databases (notably the UK Clinical Practice Research Datalink and Danish national registries) are increasingly being used to link mother and baby records to investigate the outcomes of medicines taken in pregnancy. However, some effects of drugs on the unborn baby (e.g. developmental problems) may not be detectable through databases, and may require bespoke longer term studies.

Monitoring the Safety of Biological Medicines

Scientific developments in molecular biology and genetics have been exponential since the late 1980s/early 1990s and many new active substances now reaching the market are 'biological' products which have been developed using these new technologies. Key examples include inhibitors of specific growth factors (e.g. vascular endothelial growth factor inhibitors for macular degeneration) and immunomodulators for autoimmune diseases or cancer therapy. Biological products such as erythropoietins and interferons, can (like vaccines) be prone to batch problems and minor changes in manufacturing can lead to significant clinical adverse effects. In recent years, many 'biosimilar' drugs have been developed and authorised, but these are not analogous to generic medicines and post-authorisation safety studies will be needed as part of the risk management plan.

These developments have resulted in clinical advances for many patients, but also provide new challenges for monitoring safety. Use of registries to collect information on the exposed population (see Chapter 3) may be a useful pharmacovigilance tool to study these specialised products, but better ways of accessing data and performing comparative studies are still required.

Pharmacogenetics and 'Personalised Medicine'

The discipline of pharmacogenetics is based on the premise that genetic markers can predict the safety of many drugs, with potential implications for their practical use. To date, pharmacogenetics research has mostly been focused on genetic variations in hepatic drug metabolism and on identifying hypersensitivity phenotypes. An example is the investigation of abacavir hypersensitivity, which was found to be associated with HLA-B5701. Testing was introduced in HIV clinics in London which resulted in decrease in abacavir hypersensivity from 8% to 2%. Another example is carbamazepine-induced cutaneous reactions which were found to be associated with HLA-B1502, which is more common in Asian patients. In Hong Kong, testing was recommended before prescription of carbamazepine, but some physicians saw this as an obstacle to prescribing this medicine and starting prescribing other drugs. This demonstrates how pharmacogenetics research has shown potential to identify specific patients at risk of ADRs, but also how in clinical practice there have been issues with the uptake of genetic testing. There may be several reasons for this, including costs, access to such tests and practicalities around performing such tests before prescribing a particular medicine.

The ultimate goal of pharmacogenetics research is that, in the future, ADRs could be preventable through recording of personal pharmacogenetic profiles, individual recommendations for use or avoidance of drugs, or tailored dosage regimens, for patients with specific genotypes This concept of 'personalised medicine' is both exciting and challenging for the future. It has been argued that progress has been slower than expected but, in 2015, an editorial in the *British Medical Journal* suggested that pharmacogenetics was beginning to deliver some of its potential.

Development of Scientific Methods for Pharmacovigilance Practice

Throughout this book we have touched on how scientific methods are being applied to study the safety of medicines. There have been key developments in the methods used for signal detection, prescription event monitoring and in other pharmacoepidemiology studies (see Chapter 3). Robust scientific method should be at the heart of pharmacovigilance and pharmacoepidemiology research – this is possible in many different settings around the world, but requires constant attention and review. In future clinical studies there should be more focus on patient safety as a primary end-point. This will generate valuable data on which to make benefit–risk assessments. For publication of research papers in scientific journals, peer review is now an essential part of the process and there is an almost universal requirement to report any conflicts of interest and state if ethical approval was obtained (see Chapter 8).

There remains much potential for international collaborative research, including using large datasets; global tissue banks (especially for genetic research on rare diseases or ADRs) and sharing and pooling data and expertise. Finally, there should continue to be scientific analysis, discussion and communication of results in appropriate environments, such as conferences and international meetings.

A Scientific Model for the Process of Pharmacovigilance

In terms of the overall process of pharmacovigilance, in 2003 a scientific model to support excellence in the discipline was proposed by Waller and Evans (Figure 9.1). The model represented a long-term vision of how pharmacovigilance could be conducted in the future and was underpinned by the following key concepts:

- Pharmacovigilance should be less focused on finding harm and more on extending knowledge of safety.
- There should be a clear starting point or 'specification' of what is already known at the time of licensing a medicine and what is required to extend safety knowledge post-authorisation.
- Complex risk–benefit decisions are amenable to, and likely to be improved by, the use of formal decision analysis.
- A new approach to provision of safety information which allows greater flexibility in presenting key messages based on multiple levels of information with access determined by user requirements.

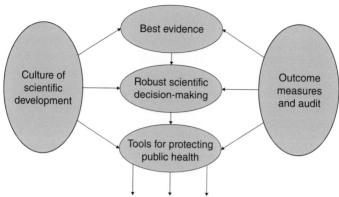

Measurable performance in terms of public health benefit

Figure 9.1 Model for excellence in pharmacovigilance.

- Flexible decision support is the most likely means of changing the behaviour of health professionals in order to promote safer use of medicines.
- There is a need to put in place outcome measures that indicate the success or failure of the process.
- Systematic audit of pharmacovigilance processes and outcomes should be developed and implemented based on agreed standards.
- Pharmacovigilance should operate in a culture of scientific development. This requires the right balance of inputs from various disciplines, a strong academic base, adequate training and resource which is dedicated to scientific strategy.

Some progress in these directions has since been made over the past decade. This includes the development of risk management plans which include a safety specification (see Chapter 5), and there has been research into the use of decision analysis for risk–benefit purposes and in measuring outcomes. As discussed next, there have also been significant developments in education within the discipline.

Education

A current and future challenge in any discipline is teaching the specialty to newcomers and the continuing development of those already working in the field. While years ago, the general model for those working in pharmacovigilance was an apprenticeship (i.e. 'learning on the job'), there have been several more recent developments, including training courses run within national authorities/organisations, and also internationally by professional organisations including the WHO Uppsala Monitoring Centre (WHO-UMC) and International Society of Pharmacovigilance (ISoP) (see Chapters 6 and 10). In some universities, pharmacovigilance is taught in the undergraduate curriculum for health sciences and there are good reasons to increase such opportunities in the future.

There are also postgraduate courses and diplomas in pharmacovigilance and pharmacoepidemiology in some countries (see Chapter 10) and online learning is now well-established. As a further measure, a collaboration between the WHO and ISoP has developed a proposed Pharmacovigilance Curriculum as a way of standardising teaching. It can be argued that the future of any specialty lies in the ability to teach it to the next generation and thus education needs remain a priority for those working in pharmacovigilance.

Public Health and Policy

It is recognised that pharmacovigilance is a key component of public health and that ADRs cause a significant clinical burden on individuals and systems around the world (see Chapter 7). Within governmental public health systems, there are several areas relevant to drug safety, the most important being the agencies or departments that regulate the quality, efficacy and safety of medicines (see Chapters 5 and 6). Here, we briefly consider recent developments and possible future directions in key public health areas.

Regulation

In the past, regulation of pharmaceuticals was much stronger before authorisation than after it. This was understandable and to some extent was appropriate, but the need for stronger regulation post-authorisation has now been recognised. In Europe, significant changes were made to regulatory legislation in 2012, which resulted in many measures to strengthen post-marketing pharmacovigilance practice (see Chapter 5). These included ways to strengthen regulation (e.g. by pan-European committees and GVP guidance documents) increase efficiency and collaboration with industry (e.g. by clarifying and streamlining processes for ADR reporting, PSURs and RMPs) and also by increasing transparency in regulatory systems. A particular challenge regulators continue to face is ways to improve systems for monitoring the safety of drugs that are authorised early on limited data (e.g. novel treatments for cancer, orphan drugs).

While there is international variation in regulatory pharmacovigilance practice around the world, many countries now use European guidance, in addition to that originating from other international organisations (see Chapter 6) and in their own country. At the time of writing (mid-2016) it appears that the UK is going to leave the EU, but we expect that medicines regulation will continue to be a collaborative process across many countries, both inside and outside the EU. It is generally agreed that the future of regulation lies in global collaboration and some ongoing international initiatives are discussed in Chapter 6.

Other Areas of Public Health

Pharmacovigilance features in several areas of public health policy; for example, in mental health policy, women's health (including family planning), hospital management and drug funding/health economics. In the future, in part due to demographic change (i.e. an increasingly older population), use of medicines is likely to increase and so the importance of pharmacovigilance in all these areas is likely to grow. Some years ago, the WHO stated that increasing access to medicines must be accompanied by appropriate systems to monitor their safety. This remains true and governmental public health policies must respond to these needs. While situations can vary from country to country, here are some suggestions for common future directions:

- Drug safety should be placed higher on the public health agenda to reflect the burden on individuals' health and on health systems.
- More government support is needed for pharmacovigilance monitoring and research, especially for prevention of ADRs.
- There should be less separation of the different 'silos' in pharmacovigilance practice (i.e. regulation, industry, science and research, patient groups, clinical practitioners) and a more collaborative and integrated means of working together alongside related sectors (e.g. health technology assessment and health economics).

- There should be ongoing public engagement of patients in ADR reporting and involvement of lay members at key stages of the pharmacovigilance process.
- There remains a need for even greater transparency in every area of pharmacovigilance practice.
- Communication is a key component of public health policy and we should continue to explore different methods to suit specific target audiences for drug safety issues. In this regard, the increasing use of social media over the past decade represents an opportunity for the future.

Conclusions

In this chapter, we have tried to give a high-level glimpse of the possible future directions of pharmacovigilance. We have considered several important areas, including improving the collection of safety data; biological medicines and pharmacogenetics; and developing and applying scientific methodology. We have also reviewed a suggested model for excellence in the pharmacovigilance process, considered education and teaching and made some suggestions for future public health policy. The next and final chapter summarises how the newcomer can deepen their knowledge, enabling them to contribute to meeting the challenges outlined.

10

Learning More About Pharmacovigilance

In the previous chapters we have generally not included specific references so as to encourage the reader to continue to learn broadly about pharmacovigilance rather than becoming too concerned about details. We also assumed that, if there were specific topics to find out more about, readers would easily be able to do so by searching the internet and/or published scientific literature. In this chapter we aim to help the newcomer who has read this far, and we hope now has some breadth of knowledge about pharmacovigilance, to approach how to deepen it.

Books

This book was originally written because there were no small books on the subject but several large ones. The large textbooks that we would recommend are as follows.

Mann's Pharmacovigilance, 3rd edition, 2014
(eds Andrews and Moore)

This is a large multi-author text with 53 chapters in five sections covering signal detection and analysis, including the use of population-based databases and pharmacoepidemiological methodologies to proactively monitor for and assess safety signals. It includes chapters on drug safety practice in specific organ classes, special populations and special products, and new developments in the field.

An Introduction to Pharmacovigilance, Second Edition. Patrick Waller and Mira Harrison-Woolrych.
© 2017 John Wiley & Sons Ltd. Published 2017 by John Wiley & Sons Ltd.

Pharmacoepidemiology, 5th edition, 2012 (eds Strom, Kimmel and Hennessy)

This has become the standard text on the subject. There is also an abridged, paperback version called *Textbook of Pharmacoepidemiology*.

Stephens' Detection and Evaluation of Adverse Drug Reactions, 6th edition, 2012 (eds Talbot and Aronson)

This book has broader scope than the title suggests and covers pharmacovigilance from industry, academic and regulatory perspectives.

Cobert's Manual of Drug Safety and Pharmacovigilance, 2nd edition, 2011

This is a very practical book with an American focus.

In terms of reference books about the adverse effects of specific drugs, the following are generally the first places to go.

Meyler's Side Effects of Drugs, 16th edition, 2015 (ed. Aronson)

Authoritative and well-referenced, if this is not in the library you use, then it should be.

Martindale: The Complete Drug Reference, 38th edition, 2014 (ed. Brayfield)

Broader in scope than *Meyler's*, if you need to find out about any drug and its adverse effects, this is a good place to start.

In terms of books on special populations, we would recommend the following texts.

Prescribing for Elderly Patients, 2009 (eds Jackson and Jansen)

This is a large practical book covering the drugs used to treat the most important clinical problems occurring the elderly.

Drugs in Pregnancy and Lactation: A Reference Guide to Fetal and Neonatal Risk, 10th edition, 2015 (eds Briggs and Freeman)

This is comprehensive reference book, with each drug monograph summarising potential side effects on the embryo and fetus and drug passage to the nursing infant.

Medicines for Women, 2015 (ed. Harrison-Woolrych)

This book is divided into three parts covering: (i) general principles of prescribing medicines for women including in pregnancy and breastfeeding; (ii) benefits and risks of specific medicine groups for women including contraceptive products, menopausal hormone therapy, bisphosphonates, human papilloma virus vaccines and herbal products; and (iii) broader perspectives including issues in developing countries and risk communication.

British National Formulary for Children

This is the essential reference guide for prescribing in children, an update of which is published annually.

Journals

Quite a few important papers in the field, including the findings of major studies, are published in the major weekly general medical journals such as the *New England Journal of Medicine, The Lancet, British Medical Journal* and *JAMA*. It is therefore a good idea to screen the contents of these titles and also the major clinical pharmacology journals. In terms of specialist journals in the field of pharmacovigilance, the two major titles, both of which appear monthly, are:

- *Drug Safety* This is the official journal of International Society of Pharmacovigilance (IsoP) (publishing all conference abstracts) and also publishes themed editions, for example on risk communication.
- *Pharmacoepidemiology and Drug Safety* This journal regularly includes a section called 'current awareness' which lists recent literature relevant to drug safety.

Another journal which is very useful in that respect is *Reactions Weekly* which is primarily an alerting service based on case reports, but also covers topical issues and news in the field.

All these journals are available in both paper and electronic formats and access is essential for anyone working in the field.

The Internet

We have mentioned and provided the addresses of some key websites for pharmacovigilance in Boxes 5.1 and 6.1. In particular, the websites of the WHO-UMC and the major regulatory agencies are worth visiting for information about specific issues/alerts, bulletins and to obtain ADR data. While official websites generally provide reliable information on pharmacovigilance, we would like to add a word of caution about searching the internet for data on drug safety issues. It is worth remembering that anyone can set up a website and – as there is no regulation of information posted on the internet – some content may therefore be misleading and/or promotional.

Courses

Opportunities for training in the field are increasing all time and it is impossible to be comprehensive here. We are aware of a variety of options in many countries. In the UK, basic courses are run by the Drug Safety Research Unit and there are also courses at certificate level (e.g. at the London School of Hygiene), and diploma and masters level (e.g. at the Universities of Hertfordshire and Portsmouth). In Europe, there is a programme known as EU2P (European Programme in Pharmacovigilance and Pharmacoepidemiology) which offers a variety of courses at all levels, including the opportunity to undertake distance learning online. Training courses are also run by the two international societies mentioned below and by the WHO-UMC. Training materials and courses regarding the use of the Medical Dictionary for Regulatory Activities (MedDRA) are available via their website.

International Societies

Finally, there are two professional societies which exist to promote development, training and international collaboration in their disciplines:

- International Society of Pharmacovigilance (ISoP)
- International Society for Pharmacoepidemiology (ISPE).

See Chapter 6 for further information about these societies.

Final Conclusions

The overarching messages we would like the newcomer to take away from this book are that pharmacovigilance is:

1) A means of potentially preventing patients coming to harm as a result of the medicines they take in expectation of benefit through:
   - Science and research
   - Regulation and other public health policy
   - Clinical practice and post-marketing monitoring
   - Effective communication about benefit–risk of medicines.
2) A vital stage of drug development. There is a need for a medicine to be shown to be acceptably safe in clinical practice.
3) A developing discipline with a global focus and plenty of scope for innovation. One of the attractions of the field that may not be immediately obvious is that, although pharmacovigilance is a specialised subject, its application is very broad indeed. Every issue is different and there are no set recipes for dealing with the next safety concern to land on your desk.

Glossary

Absolute risk The probability of an adverse event occurring expressed in absolute terms (e.g. as a rate per thousand patients, or as a proportion). An absolute risk provides information about how frequent an event is, but makes no comparison with alternatives (see **relative risk**).

Additional monitoring A scheme for focusing attention on the safety of specific medicines introduced by the European Medicines Agency in 2013, which is primarily used for new drugs and usually lasts for 5 years after first authorisation. These products are identified by a **black triangle** symbol in the product information.

Adverse drug reaction (ADR) An *unintended and noxious effect* that is attributable to a medicine when it has been given within the normal range of doses used in humans whether or not it has been used within the terms of a marketing authorisation.

Adverse event (AE) An undesirable occurrence that occurs in the context of drug treatment but which *may or may not* be causally related to a medicine.

Bias Any process that leads to systematic distortion of results away from the truth. Many types of bias have been described so when designing a study steps usually need to be taken to eliminate or minimise bias.

Black Triangle scheme A scheme introduced in the UK in the 1980s to promote intensive surveillance of new drugs. An inverted black triangle is displayed on all product information as a reminder to health professionals to report all suspected ADRs.

An Introduction to Pharmacovigilance, Second Edition. Patrick Waller and Mira Harrison-Woolrych.
© 2017 John Wiley & Sons Ltd. Published 2017 by John Wiley & Sons Ltd.

The period of intensive surveillance is usually at least 2 years. The EU introduced a similar scheme in 2013 (see **additional monitoring**).

Case–control study A study that starts by identifying cases of the disease of interest (in this context usually a potential ADR) and makes comparisons of their past 'exposures' (e.g. to drugs) with those of controls who did not develop the disease.

Clinical trial An interventional study (e.g. of a drug treatment) conducted in patients with a specific disease or condition. Such studies usually involve comparison with placebo or other treatment and a randomisation process is used to determine allocation of treatments. Ideally, trials also blind patients and clinicians (i.e. they are double-blind) to treatment allocations. Conducting a clinical trial for research purposes requires informed consent from each patient and ethical committee approval is essential.

Cohort study A study that starts by identifying a particular population with a common characteristic (e.g. a cohort based on use of a specific drug) and follows them forward in time until some individuals have developed the outcome of interest (e.g. ADR or disease).

Confounding Distortion that occurs when measuring an association between an exposure and an outcome because a confounding factor (e.g. age) is present which influences both the probability of being exposed and the risk of the outcome occurring (see Figure 2.1).

Core (or reference) clinical safety information This is a minimum standard of safety information which is considered essential for safe use of a medicine and should be included in all product information worldwide. The concept was originally proposed by the CIOMS III working group and now constitutes an Annex to the **Periodic Safety Update Report**.

Disproportionality A statistical indication of a signal in spontaneous ADR data meaning that more reports of a specific drug–ADR combination have been received than would have been expected as 'background noise'.

Drug interaction Interference of a medicine with another substance (usually another drug) that affects the activity of either drug when both are administered together.

Large simple trial A randomised trial which, in the context of pharmacovigilance, may be useful for assessing safety. The key elements are a large sample size meaning that relative rare outcome(s) can be studied; one or very few easily measurable outcomes (e.g. mortality); and that the trial should represent the 'real world' as far as possible.

Medical Dictionary for Regulatory Activities (MedDRA) The most widely used standardised international dictionary of medical terminology for regulatory communication and evaluation of data relating to human medicines. MedDRA was developed through ICH and its use for coding is mandatory in the EU.

Medication error A failure in the treatment process that leads to, or has the potential to lead to, harm to the patient – for example, prescription of the wrong drug or giving an incorrect dose.

Meta-analysis A meta-analysis brings together data from several different studies in a quantitative way, so as to provide a single overall estimate of a specified effect. It is, in effect, a 'study of studies.'

Observational study A study in which there is no intervention in relation to the management of patients or participants. Observational research is often based on data derived from ordinary medical practice.

Orphan drug A drug used in the treatment of an 'orphan' (i.e. rare) disease. Because development may be uneconomic, incentives to companies may be provided. They are often authorised 'early' because of a lack of suitable alternative treatments and on the basis of small clinical trial programmes.

Patient Information Leaflet A summary of the product information for patients/carers, which in many countries is included in the medicine's packaging, or given to the patient as the time of dispensing. Also known the package leaflet in the EU, package insert in the USA and consumer information in some other countries.

Periodic Safety Update Report (PSUR) A systematic review of the *global* safety data which became available to the manufacturer of a marketed drug during a specified time period in an internationally agreed format. Submission of PSURs to regulatory authorities is a legal obligation in many countries.

Pharmacoepidemiology The scientific discipline of studying drug effects in populations.

Pharmacogenetics The investigation and use of genetic markers to maximise the safety and/or efficacy of drugs.

Pharmacovigilance The science and activities relating to the detection, assessment, understanding and prevention of adverse effects or any other drug-related problems (this is the current definition of the World Health Organization.

Pharmacovigilance plan This is the second part of a **risk management plan** for a medicine. The plan should indicate what pharmacovigilance activities (both routine and any additional ones that are specific to the product) will be undertaken in order to further assess its safety.

Post-authorisation safety study (PASS) A study of an authorised and marketed medicine that aims to characterise or quantify a safety hazard, assess its safety profile in real life use or measure the effectiveness of risk minimisation measures.

Post-marketing surveillance (PMS) Safety-related activity after a product is marketed. This process includes, but is not limited to, spontaneous ADR reports and specific post-marketing studies (see **post-authorisation safety study**) including **prescription-event monitoring**. After marketing, this term may be regarded as synonymous with **pharmacovigilance**.

Pre-clinical studies Studies conducted in laboratory animals; these are normally performed before initiating a clinical trial programme.

Pregnancy prevention programme An additional risk minimisation measure aimed at preventing fetal exposure to teratogenic medicines.

Prescription-event monitoring (PEM) (also known as cohort-event monitoring) A pharmacoepidemiological study in which a cohort of users of a medicine is identified from prescriptions and followed-up for a defined period to identify all adverse events occurring in the post-treatment period.

Registry A registry is a collection of individual patient data which can be used for epidemiological studies and can based on a disease, treatment, specific exposure or outcome.

Relative risk The probability of an adverse event occurring expressed in relative terms against a specified comparator. A relative risk provides information about the strength of an association, but it does not indicate how common or rare an event is in absolute terms (see **absolute risk**).

Risk–benefit balance All medicines have both risks and benefits, and for their use to be acceptable the balance of these must be judged to favour benefit. Making the judgement requires consideration of all the relevant data and this can be summarised in a benefit–risk report.

Risk management plan (RMP) A document prepared by a pharmaceutical company specifying what is and what is not known about the safety of a product, what is planned to extend safety knowledge and how known risks will be minimised.

Risk minimisation Measures designed to minimise the occurrence of known ADRs. These are outlined in a risk minimisation plan which is the final part of a **risk management plan**.

Safety Relative absence of harm. When we say that a drug is 'safe', we mean that there is a low probability of harm that, *in the context of the disease being treated and the expected benefits of the drug*, can be considered acceptable.

Safety specification This is the first part of a **risk management plan** which considers the evidence for and level of safety that has been demonstrated so far. The specification should identify both what is and what *is not* yet known about safety.

Seriousness An ADR or case report should be considered 'serious' if it meets any of the following criteria:
- Fatal outcome
- Life-threatening
- Led to or prolonged hospitalisation
- Led to long-term disability
- Congenital abnormality.

In addition, it is possible for a case to be medically judged as serious even if none of the above criteria are met.

Severity The degree of impact of a particular ADR in an individual patient (usually subjective and judged by the patient or doctor) which is often categorised as mild, moderate or severe. This concept is distinct from **seriousness**, and it is possible to have an ADR that is severe (e.g. a very bad headache) but which does not meet the criteria for seriousness.

Side effect An unintended effect of a medicine.

Signal An alert requiring further investigation from any available data source that a drug *may* be associated with a previously unrecognised hazard. The term is also used when there is new evidence that a known hazard *may* be quantitatively (e.g. more frequent) or qualitatively (e.g. more serious) different from what was previously known.

Spontaneous ADR report A case report relating to an individual patient describing a *suspected* adverse reaction.

Summary of Product Characteristics (SPC or SmPC) A regulatory document in the EU which is attached to the marketing authorisation which forms the basis of the product information (as it is more widely known) and is primarily directed at prescribers.

Systematic review A systematic review evaluates all the relevant research relating to a particular question. The Cochrane Collaboration uses this method to appraise medical treatments and publishes its findings in the Cochrane Library.

Yellow Card scheme The UK national spontaneous ADR reporting scheme. In some other countries, spontaneous reporting schemes also use yellow reporting cards, although electronic forms are now becoming more common.

Index

Page numbers in **bold** refer to Tables; those in *italics* refer to Figures

An Introduction to Pharmacovigilance, Second Edition. Patrick Waller
and Mira Harrison-Woolrych.
© 2017 John Wiley & Sons Ltd. Published 2017 by John Wiley & Sons Ltd.